An RNID Handbook

YOUR HEARING LOSS
and how to cope with it

KENNETH LYSONS

DAVID & CHARLES
Newton Abbot　London　North Pomfret (Vt)　Vancouver

To Audrey, Michael, Jeffrey and Edith

British Library Cataloguing in Publication Data
Lysons, Kenneth
  Your hearing loss.
  1. Hearing disorder
  I. Title
  617.8′02′408162   RF290   77–85015

ISBN 0–7153–7472–9

Library of Congress Catalog Card Number: 77-85015

© Kenneth Lysons 1978

All rights reserved. No part of this
publication may be reproduced, stored
in a retrieval system, or transmitted,
in any form or by any means, electronic,
mechanical, photocopying, recording or
otherwise, without the prior permission
of David & Charles (Holdings) Limited

Set by G. C. Typeset Limited, Bolton, Greater Manchester
and printed in Great Britain
by Biddles Limited, Guildford
for David & Charles (Holdings) Limited
Brunel House, Newton Abbot, Devon

Published in the United States of America
by David & Charles Inc.
North Pomfret Vermont 05053 USA

Published in Canada
by Douglas David & Charles Limited
1875 Welch Street North Vancouver BC

Contents

	INTRODUCTION	5
1	AN EXPERIENCE OF HEARING LOSS	8
2	THE MECHANISM OF HEARING	12
	the outer ear . the middle ear . the inner ear . how the mechanism works	
3	SOME CAUSES OF HEARING LOSS	18
	the nature of hearing loss . the causes of hearing loss . tinnitus	
4	MEASURING HEARING AND HEARING LOSS	27
	sound and decibels . audiometers and audiometry . taking an audiometric test . the measurement of hearing handicap . interpreting audiograms	
5	YOU AND YOUR OTOLOGIST	45
	visiting the otologist . how the otologist makes his diagnosis . what can the otologist do?	
6	HEARING IMPAIRMENT IS MORE THAN DULL EARS	56
	how and why emotions and behaviour are affected . coping with the effects	
7	HEARING AIDS AND OTHER DEVICES	66
	types of hearing aids . their components . the National Health aid and how to get one . commercial aids . buying a commercial aid . consumer protection and the hearing-aid user . the use and maintenance of an aid . other aids to hearing	
8	LIPREADING	87
	the basis of lipreading . its limitations and advantages . learning to lipread . lipreading in practice . supplementing lipreading . auditory training	

9	EMPLOYMENT, LEISURE AND FAMILY RELATIONSHIPS	102
10	STATUTORY AND VOLUNTARY SERVICES	114

APPENDICES
I Hearing Aid Council Code of Practice 121
II Useful Organisations 124

ACKNOWLEDGEMENTS 126

INDEX 127

Introduction

This book is intended for anyone who is hard of hearing or deafened, or thinks he or she will become so; for anyone who lives or works with people who have impaired hearing; and for all who wish to know something about hearing disability and how it may be helped.

Three categories are covered by the generic term 'hearing-impaired': the hard of hearing, the deafened and the deaf. Since in ordinary speech we use the word 'deaf' to cover all three types of hearing impairment, whatever its cause, age of onset or severity, it is useful at the outset to distinguish between 'the deaf' and 'the hard of hearing'.

The deaf are the people whose sense of hearing is non-functional for the ordinary purposes of life. People in this category have no *usable* hearing. Some are *congenitally deaf*, either born deaf or becoming deaf before acquiring speech; the others are '*deafened*' or '*adventitiously deaf*', meaning that their sense of hearing became non-functional later in life, probably through disease or accident.

The hard of hearing are those people in whom the sense of hearing, although defective, is functional with or without a hearing aid.

People *born* deaf are excluded from this book for three reasons. Firstly, their problems are different from those of the hard of hearing and the deafened. The lifelong handicap that a person born without usable hearing has to overcome is the difficulty of acquiring adequate speech and language. A child who becomes profoundly deaf at, say, the age of seven will have acquired speech, vocabulary and language pattern in a natural way, by hearing words used in conversation and perceiving their meanings in different contexts. In contrast, the born-deaf child is 'deaf, dumb and wordless' (I. R. and A. W. G. Ewing, *Opportunity and the Deaf Child*). Until specially instructed by specialist teachers, his manner of expressing himself will be limited to gestures and unintelligible sounds. To use a somewhat crude analogy, a deaf child is in a similar position to that of a person who has to learn a foreign language before he can be taught any other subject. To quote J. D. Evans,

> Between the psychological attitudes of the deaf and the deafened (or hard of hearing) there is an almost unbridgeable gulf. It must be emphasised that at the beginning of their lives the deaf are abnormals shut off from that stream of verbally conveyed ideas which moulds the individual mind to general sameness with the mental pattern of society and throughout their lives the deaf are abnormals struggling towards full normalcy. The deafened on the other hand are normals threatened with all the horror of abnormalcy. To the change in their state and particularly the change in the behaviour of other people towards them they are particularly sensitive . . . they will not class themselves with the 'true deaf' nor will they approach deaf organisations for help. They are thus a class apart. ('Voluntary Organisations for the Welfare of the Deaf' in *Voluntary Social Services – Their Place in the Modern State*, Methuen.)

Thirdly, the born deaf are fortunately much fewer in number than the hard of hearing. In 1951 the then Ministry of Health estimated that there was about one deaf person to every 2,000 of the population. In 1973, 25,900 deaf and 18,800 hard of hearing were on the registers which local authorities are required to keep under Section 29 of the National Assistance Act 1948. These figures are certainly understatements, particularly of the numbers of the hard of hearing, since not everyone eligible to register does so. In 1947 the Social Survey Division of the Central Office of Information made a survey for the Medical Research Council to ascertain the numbers of government hearing aids likely to be required under the National Health Service Act passed in the previous year. It was based on a stratified random sample of the civilian populations aged sixteen years and over in England, Scotland and Wales. Hearing ability was defined in seven categories:

CATEGORY	TERM	CRITERIA	NUMBERS
7	Deaf mutes	Those who became deaf in early life and who learned speech by special means	15,000

CATEGORY	TERM	CRITERIA	NUMBERS
6	Totally deaf	Person cannot hear speech at all but had learned speech by normal means before becoming deaf	30,000
5	Deaf to all natural speech	Person has difficulty in hearing loudly spoken speech but can hear amplified speech by means of a hearing aid or trumpet	70,000
4	Hard of hearing	Person has difficulty in hearing normal direct speech but can hear loudly spoken speech	790,000
3	Hard of hearing	Person has difficulty in hearing in any part of a theatre or church or in group conversation, but can hear speech at short range without aid	860,000
			1,765,000

Categories 1 and 2 referred respectively to those who 'can hear all normal speech in any part of theatre/church without aid' and 'have one defective ear but can hear all normal speech in any part of church or theatre without aid'. Other estimates are that one in three of the adult population has some degree of hearing loss, though not necessarily of sufficient severity to require the use of an aid or to constitute a disability.

It is therefore for everyone with an acquired hearing impairment that this book is written.

1 An Experience of Hearing Loss

In 1941, at the age of 18, I stood at one end of a long room with my right ear blocked by an orderly while I repeated words whispered by an Air Force medical officer standing some twenty feet away. 'Tomato,' he whispered. 'Tomato,' I responded. 'Disaster.' 'Disaster,' I echoed obediently. 'Nothing wrong there,' said the MO, 'We'll try the other ear.' Out of the corner of my eye I saw him mouthing words but to my surprise I was unable to hear what he was saying. He came closer and closer but not until he was only about six feet away was I able to repeat the words with any confidence. The medical officer inflated my ear without any improvement; he tested my bone and air conduction with tuning forks, finally he gave his verdict. 'You are suffering from a condition of the middle ear which will get worse and which flying might aggravate. I am recommending you for discharge. When you get out see an ear specialist immediately otherwise you may, in time, become stone deaf.'

I protested that I heard conversation without difficulty and didn't feel in the least deaf but he was adamant and at last I staggered blindly out of the room. What I thought was no more than a routine 'medical' to establish my fitness for flying duties had altered the whole outlook of my life.

Some weeks later I saw an eminent otologist and my doctor gave me a copy of his report. Certain phrases of that letter burnt themselves into my memory: 'This young man is suffering from otosclerotic deafness which will get worse. We know of no cure for it. . . . It is difficult to suggest an occupation in which he will not be handicapped although farming should be a suitable calling for a deaf person. . . . He will doubtless find it difficult to adjust himself to his disability.'

My hearing deteriorated insidiously rather than dramatically and it was almost six years after the discovery of the impairment before I had to use a hearing aid. Feeling too young to be deaf, and that wearing a hearing aid would only advertise my disability, I resorted to all kinds of subterfuges to give the impression of having normal hearing. When shopping I always tried to tender a pound note for purchases worth less to avoid the embarrassment of having to admit that I had not heard the price of an article. I insisted on walking so that my best ear was turned towards my companion. If all else failed I made vague references to having a 'heavy cold' which had 'bunged up' my eustachian tubes. Like many hard of hearing people I began to shun company and increasingly devoted myself to solitary pursuits.

In the meantime I had started a job and married. In spite of the telephone I was happy at work because my colleagues in the office had soon discovered that my hearing was faulty, and I could give up pretending. My home life was a relief from the strain of the outside world and at the end of the day I found much joy in reading and in music, particularly Bach's organ works to which I listened with two hearing aids, a commercial aid in one ear and the government aid in the other, and when alone, with the volume control of the record player turned full on.

As I became more accustomed to the role of a hard-of-hearing person my attitude became less rebellious and more constructive. I recognized that if I was to hold my own in the field of employment I had to be not only good at my job but also better qualified than the next man. Realizing also that a change of occupation might be necessary, I resolved to do two things: firstly, to be as informed as possible about hearing impairment and how it could be helped; secondly, to improve my qualifications and cultivate interests that could be remunerative should I ever be forced to relinquish normal employment. In the evenings therefore, instead of engaging in desultory reading, I began to study for specific examinations. The hearing loss was a help here rather than a hindrance since, in the winter evenings, I could work by the fire with my hearing aid turned off while my wife could watch television without distracting me. After three or four years I had obtained some recognized qualifications, including those of the Chartered Institute of Secretaries, a Diploma in Management Studies and five Advanced Level GCEs; I was also halfway to an accountancy qualification. Initially the motivation was that my 'bits of paper' would be a form of insurance against unsuitable employment. If the worst came to the worst I could run an accountancy practice at home, act as tutor for a correspondence college and engage in spare-time journalism. Later, the discovery that I could pass examinations had the effect of restoring my self-confidence, thus helping to compensate for feelings of inferiority.

One result of obtaining qualifications, however, was the wish to find a responsible job which would use my knowledge. Obtaining interviews for more senior jobs was easy enough, but I sensed that most employers wrote me off directly they saw my hearing aid. Some actually tried to test my hearing by speaking abnormally softly.

One day I saw an advertisement offering a one-year course of training to would-be teachers in technical colleges. Cold reason told me that I would be rejected on medical grounds, but more in hope than confidence I filled in the application forms. At that time I was wearing an aid with an invisi-mould and perhaps the interviewing committee did not notice it. At any rate they accepted me. I had a wonderful year in the college, becoming President of the Union and obtaining my teacher's certificate with a distinction. Unfortunately, at the end of the course there was a medical examination conducted by a doctor from the then Ministry of Education who refused to let me wear my aid and turned me down as medically unfit for teaching. I now fought a battle royal with the Ministry, in which I was supported most nobly by the college principal who travelled to London to plead my cause. Eventually, the Ministry relented and I was recognized as a qualified teacher.

Subject to such recognition I had obtained a post as an assistant lecturer at a college near my home. Most of my classes were small and I coped without too much difficulty. The work was rewarding, especially in the opportunities it provided for helping students to progress in their own careers. Further advance in the teaching profession demanded a university degree, however, and by teaching five evenings weekly, and in one year on a Saturday morning, I was able to have sufficient time off in the day to attend a university eight miles away. Eventually I obtained my diploma with first-class passes in all but one subject and was encouraged to proceed to an MA, and subsequently to MEd and PhD degrees.

At this point I recalled my earlier resolve to know as much as possible about hearing impairment, telling myself 'Your hearing is progressively deteriorating, why not look at what is being done for the welfare of the deaf?' For my thesis 'Some Aspects of the Historical Development and Present Organisation of Voluntary

Welfare Societies for Adult Deaf Persons in England 1840–1963' I was more than fortunate in the co-operation I received. Dr Pierre Gorman, then librarian of the Royal National Institute for the Deaf, was tireless in his help; over 80 per cent of welfare officers replied to my questionnaires; the RNID awarded me a travelling scholarship and I could thus spend vacations visiting welfare societies, schools and other centres of work for the deaf and meeting many people with specialist knowledge of hearing impairment.

Surgical procedures were then being developed for the treatment of middle-ear deafness. These are described in Chapter 5. I hesitated about the fenestration operation and decided to wait until the results were more permanent. A stapes mobilization was unsuccessful but I decided to try again with a stapedectomy; the results exceeded my wildest dreams. I was able both to discard my aid and hear naturally without strain. I was so delighted with the result of the first stapedectomy on my left ear that a year later I had the right ear treated and again obtained a very significant improvement in hearing. Ten years later (1976) the second result is as good as ever. The left ear has lost some acuity but is still serviceable, especially for the telephone. Every day I am thankful that it is no longer necessary for otologists to write helplessly 'We know of no cure for it' for the vast majority of otosclerotic cases. The psychological uplift resulting from the restoration of socially adequate hearing has been tremendous.

Often during the twenty years in which I was hard of hearing I longed for a book which would deal in a simple but informed way with the main problems encountered. The purpose of this chapter is to declare my credentials for attempting to write such a book.

2 The Mechanism of Hearing

Impaired hearing concentrates the mind wonderfully on the ears, which otherwise we all take for granted. Because the ability to hear well is accepted as normal, most people have only a vague idea of the complex mechanism by which the ear performs its functions of collecting, modifying, amplifying and analysing sound. Some knowledge of this mechanism is essential, however, to understand the various forms of hearing impairment.

The ear has three parts, the outer, middle and inner ears. The contribution to hearing of each of these parts will first be considered, with reference to Fig 1.

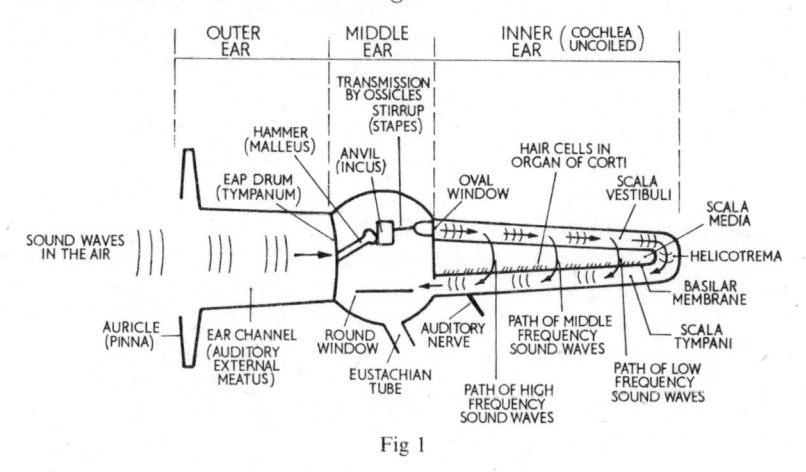

Fig 1

THE OUTER EAR

The outer ear comprises a sound receptor, known as the auricle or pinna, and an inner passage called the ear canal or the external auditory meatus. The auricle resembles a cupped hand and helps to amplify sound waves in front of the ear. When hard of hearing people place a hand behind an ear and cup the ear in the direction of a sound they are, in effect, providing an enlargement of the auricle and thus gaining further amplification.

The external meatus is a cul-de-sac, approximately 25 mm in length, which terminates at the ear drum or tympanum. The tympanum itself is a translucent cone-shaped membrane, about 10 mm in diameter and approximately the same thickness as a sheet of newspaper. Middle 'C' on a piano which is a pure tone causes the tympanum to make 256 vibrations per second but it is of interest that the ear drum's vibrations move through a distance equivalent only to the diameter of a hydrogen atom (0.000000001 mm).

THE MIDDLE EAR

Although the cavity between the inner side of the tympanum and the inner ear is very small, within this space three functions essential to the transmission of sound take place. Firstly, for a reason that will be explained later, vibrations on the tympanum are carried at increased force to the inner ear by means of a lever system consisting of three bones called the ossicles. In order of operation, the ossicles are the malleus, or hammer, which is attached to the tympanum; the incus, or anvil, and the stapes, or stirrup. The bottom part of the stirrup known as the footplate fits into an aperture in the inner ear termed the oval window. To give some idea of the minute size of the ossicles, the stapes, the smallest of the three bones, is only about 3 mm high and weighs scarcely 3 milligrams.

The second contribution made by the middle ear is to maintain an equal air pressure on each side of the tympanum. This pressure is maintained by air which reaches the middle ear through the eustachian tube. The eustachian tube leads into the middle ear from the back of the throat, and can be opened by yawning or swallowing.

Thirdly, the middle ear contains two important muscles, one attached to the tympanum, appropriately called the tensor tympani, and one connected to the stapes called the stapedius. The stapedius has the distinction of being the smallest muscle in the human body. The purpose of these muscles is to give the tympanum and the stapes an opportunity to brace themselves against very loud, low-pitched sounds and thus protect the delicate membrane in the oval window from possible rupture.

THE INNER EAR

The inner ear is responsible for the analysis of complex sound frequencies, the transduction of sound waves into nerve impulses and their subsequent transmission to the areas of the brain where they are heard as sounds. The inner ear also contains the three semi-circular canals which play no part in hearing but, together with two small sac-like chambers, the utricle and the saccule, jointly known as the vestibule, are concerned with the maintenance of balance.

The organ of hearing itself is the cochlea—the Greek word for snail, as its external appearance is very similar to the shell of a small snail. If uncoiled the $2\frac{3}{4}$ turns of the shell would form a tube about 30–35 mm long and about 5 mm in diameter. Throughout its length the cochlea is divided into two galleries, partly by a bony shelf and partly by a membrane called the basilar membrane, which varies in thickness from less than 0.001 mm near its basal end to 0.005 mm at the apex of the cochlea. These two galleries are each filled with a watery fluid called perilymph. The larger end of the upper gallery, or scala vestibuli, connects with the middle ear at the oval window, where the footplate of the stapes makes a fluid-proof seal. The lower gallery, or scala tympani, meets the middle ear at another aperture, named the round window. The two galleries communicate with each other at the apex through a gap, termed the helicotrema.

From the roof of the upper gallery, another membrane, Reissner's membrane (see Fig 2) slopes downwards to form an inner passage shaped like a right-angled triangle, and referred to as the scala media. The scala media is also filled with a fluid, endolymph. Resting on the part of the basilar membrane that forms the flow of the scala media is the organ of Corti, named after Alfrenso Corti who first discovered it in 1851. It is in the organ of Corti that the conversion of sound waves into electrical impulses takes place. Within the organ of Corti are about 23,000 hair cells, arranged in an inner row and four outer rows of rods or pillars. Near the bases of the hair cells are auditory nerve fibres, between 25,000 and 30,000 in number. Although there is just over one nerve fibre to each hair cell the relationship is not on a one-to-one basis and a nerve fibre may act like a telephone party-line in supplying endings to many hair cells. The upper ends of the hair cells pass through a thin membrane called the

Fig 2

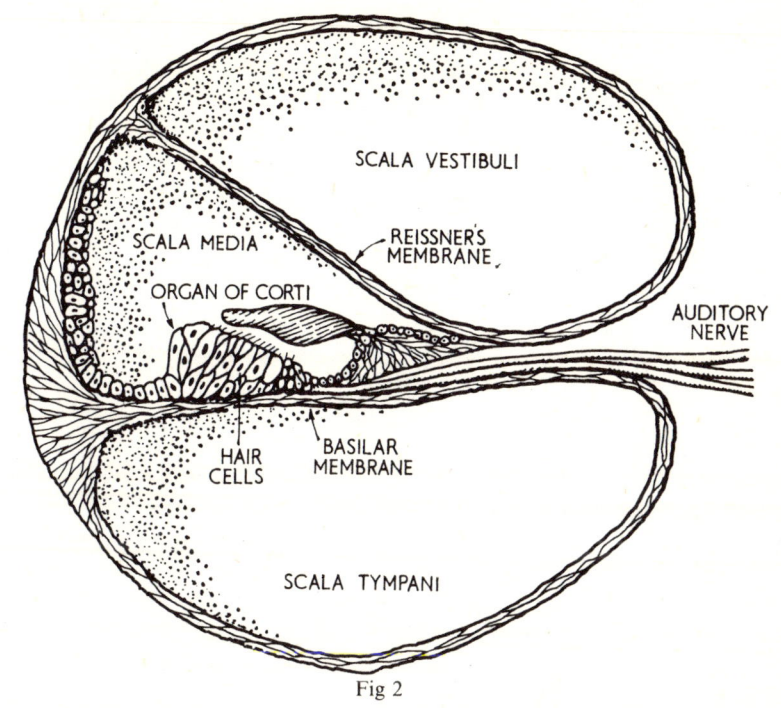

recticula lamina, and are embedded in a thicker covering membrane which lies like a flap over the organ of Corti. On leaving the cochlea these fibres twist together, rather like the strands of a rope, to form the auditory nerve which conveys the electrical impulses to the temporal portion of the brain.

HOW THE MECHANISM WORKS

Having described the physiology of the ear we can now put the three parts together to see how the mechanism works. Sound waves, which in the young adult vary in frequency from 20 to 20,000 cycles per second or hertz, are collected by the auricle and cause the tympanum to vibrate. These vibrations are conducted across the middle ear by the ossicles; they are then transmitted to the cochlea in the inner ear through the rocking of the stapes in the oval window. So far the sound waves have been transmitted through air; at the oval window they pass into fluid. As a liquid provides higher impedance than air, it follows that the sound pressure on the almost incompressible watery fluid, the perilymph, of the inner ear must be greater than in the highly compressible air of the middle ear. This increased pressure is partly provided by the lever action of the ossicles and partly by the fact that the diameter of the tympanum is about twenty times that of the footplate of the stapes, which therefore exerts twenty times the original pressure on the oval window. The action of the stapes on the oval window causes the perilymph to move over Reissner's membrane round the gap, the helicotrema, and then over the other surface of the basal membrane until it reaches the round window, which thus absorbs the pressure and acts as a kind of safety valve.

A vibration of a particular frequency results in a wave-like ripple which reaches its maximum at a given point along the basilar membrane. Thus, high-frequency sounds cause vibrations near the oval window, while low-frequency ones cause oscillations further along the whole membrane. The movement of the basilar membrane results in a shearing effect between the hair cells of the organ of Corti and the covering (tectorial) membrane; this, in some way not yet understood, causes an electro-chemical reaction in the nerve fibres. The reaction is transmitted by the auditory nerve to the brain. In the brain the information received is decoded and presented as intelligible sound. It has been estimated that the human ear can identify some 350,000 distinct sounds.

The minuteness of the whole apparatus is impressive. So is its high level of perfection. It has been stated that the ossicles of the middle ear form a mathematically perfect transmission system, while the contra-actions of the oval and round windows on the perilymph provide an ideal hydraulic system. Finally, although it has taken several pages to describe, the whole process, from the reception of sound waves by the auricle to their interpretation in the auditory cortex of the brain, takes no longer than three-hundredths of a second.

HEARING WITH BOTH EARS

Binaural hearing is the term used to describe hearing with two ears; in monaural hearing only one ear is used. Following accident or disease many people have varying degrees of impairment affecting one ear only. Where the 'good' ear is normal or nearly so they may not be greatly inconvenienced.

There are, however, a number of reasons why two functional ears are better than one. Experiments have shown that with binaural hearing sensitivity to sound is increased and, under noisy conditions, speech is more intelligible. Several researchers (see for instance S. E. Gerber, *Introducing Hearing Science*—W. B. Sanders, Philadelphia) have also observed that while the right ear is more efficient at processing speech sounds, the left ear is better with non-speech stimuli such as music. Furthermore, as all stereo enthusiasts know, binaural hearing assists in locating the direction from which a sound comes. A sound wave from a given direction may strike the ear nearest the sound source fractionally before the other. This principle was used, incidentally, in pre-radar days in a curious invention known as the Topophone or Stereophonic Direction Finder. The purpose of this device was to enable the captain or pilot of a ship to locate the direction of warning signals in foggy weather.

3 Some Causes of Hearing Loss

Anyone trying to help a person with impaired hearing must have accurate information about the type of loss and how it has arisen. How an otologist may seek such information will be described in Chapter 4. The different types of hearing impairment and some of the more common conditions that cause it are described here. Some of the ways in which the extent of the loss can be measured are outlined in Chapters 3 and 4.

THE NATURE OF HEARING LOSS

A loss of hearing may be placed in one of four categories. Firstly there are impairments that affect the outer and middle ears, resulting in a *conductive loss*. Secondly, there are conditions affecting the inner ear, which give rise to *perceptive* or *sensorineural loss*. A third type of loss, *central loss*, is not dealt with here. It can arise from a variety of causes such as brain damage or abnormalities that are mental rather than physical in origin. An example of central loss is sensory aphasia, in which a person is unable to understand the meaning of words although he has no difficulty in hearing the actual sounds. Finally there is *mixed loss*, in which the impairment is partly conductive and partly sensorineural. Apart from the tests described in Chapters 3 and 5, it is possible to make a rough assessment of whether an individual has a predominantly conductive or sensorineural loss from noting the following signs:

	CONDUCTIVE LOSS	SENSORINEURAL LOSS
TYPICAL SPEECH	Low and soft, as the person can hear his or her own voice through bone conduction	Speech is loud with a tendency to shout, as the person has difficulty in hearing his own voice

	CONDUCTIVE LOSS	SENSORINEURAL LOSS
TOLERATION OF LOUDNESS	Loud sounds and speech can be tolerated	Loud sounds and speech, of an intensity considerably above the threshold of hearing, may cause discomfort
BACKGROUND NOISE	Hearing is better in a noise	Noise may adversely affect discrimination, due to recruitment

Both conductive and sensorineural losses can be due to a wide variety of causes, some of which are set out below.

SOME CAUSES OF ACQUIRED HEARING LOSS

Conductive Loss
1. Obstructions in the outer ear, due to excessive wax or foreign bodies.
2. Accidents—blows or head injuries, damaging the ear-drum or the ossicles.
3. Infections—acute or chronic otitis-media can develop from colds, measles, tonsillitis and other infections of the nose and throat. (Secretory otitis media affects 10 per cent of all children of school age.)
4. Otosclerosis, the immobilisation of the stapes by a growth of spongy bone.

Sensorineural Loss
1. Accidents—such as fracture of the skull, etc, or exposure to explosive blasts.
2. Infections—virus infections such as mumps, or the effects of chronic otitis media or meningitis.
3. Noise—prolonged exposure to noise at above 100 decibels.
4. Ototoxic loss can be caused by ear-poisoning drugs, especially quinine and antibiotics such as streptomycin and neomycin.
5. Presbyacusis, the hearing impairment due to age.
6. Ménière's disease, which has a triad of symptoms—vertigo, tinnitus and hearing loss.
7. Miscellaneous causes, including interruption of the blood supply of the inner ear, virus infection of unknown origin, or tumours.

Four of the most common causes of hearing loss are discussed here; two being conductive and two of the sensorineural type. A brief reference is also made to tinnitus or head noises which many people with a hearing impairment find a particularly troublesome symptom.

CONDUCTIVE LOSS

Most cases of conductive hearing impairment are due either to inflammation of the middle ear (otitis-media) or to a condition known as otosclerosis.

Otitis-media
Otitis-media is a general term applied to a variety of infections of the middle ear. In its acute forms otitis-media may be due to bacteria spreading up the eustachian tube as a complication of colds, tonsilitis and similar affections of the nose and throat. It may also result from the eustachian tube not working properly possibly due to infection.

In the case of infection, invading germs cause the mucous membrane lining the middle ear to become inflamed. The inflammation causes fluid secreted in the mucous membrane to exude. If not quickly relieved by antibiotics the pressure exerted by the fluid may lead to rupturing of the ear-drum, pain, and an ear discharge. Whether the ear-drum ruptures or not, it will distend and a loss of hearing will result.

In the second case, the eustachian tube may not function properly for a number of reasons. If its lining becomes swollen due to a cold, or if it is blocked at its entrance by an enlarged adenoid, the tube is unable to perform its function of ensuring that the air pressure on the inside of the ear-drum is equal to that on the outside. The drum is therefore forced inwards and the amount of air remaining in the middle ear is gradually absorbed by the mucous membrane and replaced as fluid. Again loss of hearing results from the reduced ability of the drum and the ossicles to transmit vibrations.

Otitis-media used to be the commonest cause of acquired hearing impairment in children. There was also the danger that further complications might develop, such as the infection of the mastoid process. Today, little permanent hearing impairment results from acute otitis-media, due to the prompt use of sulphonamide drugs and antibiotics such as penicillin.

There is still the danger, however, that repeated attacks of acute otitis-media may give rise to a chronic condition. Chronic otitis-media may be suppurative or non-suppurative. One example of a non-discharging condition is chronic secretory otitis-media, which can occur after an inflammatory infection has been treated by antibiotics. The action of the drugs neutralizes the infection but the fluid, now sterile, remains in the middle ear and gradually thickens until it becomes glue-like in consistency. The thicker the glue the more the movement of the three small bones in the middle ear is impeded. If untreated the hearing may deteriorate further because of adhesions on the ossicles, or the disruption or destruction of the ossicular chain.

Chronic suppurative otitis-media may occur when a perforation in the ear-drum has become permanent, thereby providing an alternative to the eustachian tube as a route by which infections may enter the middle ear. It is for this reason that anyone with a perforated ear-drum is generally advised not to swim. The fluid discharged through the drum may be either odourless or foul smelling. The distinction is important, for while otologists regard the former as relatively harmless, the latter may be symptomatic of a potentially serious condition known as cholesteatoma of the middle ear. The cholesteatoma or cyst contains bone-eroding matter which may destroy the ossicles. If untreated the cyst grows insidiously and may invade the inner ear, changing a treatable conductive impairment into an irreversible sensorineural deafness.

Otosclerosis

Otosclerosis, a disease of the bony wall of the labyrinth, is the commonest cause of hearing impairment during the period from young adulthood up to early middle age. The term otosclerosis, meaning a hardening of the ear bone, is misleading since the effect of the disease is to replace the normal hard bone with soft spongy bone. Otosclerosis has been called a 'pathological engima'; as yet, in spite of much research, no firm conclusions on its cause have been reached.

Otosclerosis develops insidiously and may be noticed by people in their late teens or early twenties although the peak incidence occurs at about thirty years of age. The hearing loss is due to the stapes becoming fixed, or anchylosed, in the oval window because of an overgrowth of the spongy bone. At first the impairment may be slight although hearing acuity deteriorates at varying rates. (There may even be periods when the loss gets no worse.) In its later stages the disease may invade the middle ear so that the condition changes from a conductive to a mixed loss.

Otosclerosis of course shows the general indications of conductive impairment described earlier in this chapter. It also has the following characteristics:

> It is estimated to be twice as prevalent in women as in men; pregnancy may be a precipitating factor.
> There is usually, though not necessarily, a family history of 'deafness'.
> With conductive otosclerosis, bone conduction will be better than air conduction; it may be possible to hear on the telephone even when there is difficulty in hearing normal speech.
> Tinnitus is often present and in mild cases may be the most distressing symptom.
> The hearing loss usually begins in one ear, and then in most cases becomes bilateral; but the degree of hearing loss is not the same in both ears.
> Otosclerosis is more prevalent in white than in black races, and among the fair-haired.

While otitis-media and otosclerosis are the two most important causes of conductive impairment they are dissimilar in several respects. Otitis-media is a disease of childhood, although its consequences may persist through adult life. Otosclerosis becomes apparent in early adulthood. The hereditary 'deafness' that can often be traced in otosclerosis patients does not arise in otitis-media. There are also differences that can be detected only by the otologist; in otitis-media both the ear-drum and the eustachian tube show signs of abnormality, in otosclerosis they are usually normal.

SENSORINEURAL HEARING LOSS

Although sensorineural loss may occur at any stage of life it is particularly associated with birth and with the degenerative consequences of ageing. Congenital impairment is outside the scope of this book, but among the common causes of profound hearing loss at or before birth are the mother contracting rubella—German measles—during the first three months of pregnancy, rhesus incompatibility and anoxia, or lack of oxygen, causing brain damage at the time of birth. In early adulthood or middle age a condition known as Ménière's disease may be a distressing manifestation of sensorineural loss, while old age is usually accompanied by some hearing impairment.

Ménière's Disease

Ménière's disease, named after Prosper Ménière, a Paris physician who first described the condition in 1861, is a dysfunction of the inner ear. Its symptoms are intermittent attacks of vertigo accompanied by tinnitus and hearing loss.

The vertigo, which usually begins abruptly, is the most distinctive symptom and typically takes the form of a 'whirling' sensation in which the affected person feels that either he or his surroundings are 'spinning round'. It may also take the form of a sensation of going up and down or, as Ménière himself put it 'being on the bridge of a ship at the mercy of a stormy sea'. This dizziness may persist for several hours and then become quiescent for varying intervals of time which may become shorter if not treated. The vertigo is always accompanied by a feeling of nausea and actual vomiting.

Tinnitus, the second symptom, commonly takes the form of a low buzzing or hissing sound and persists after the vertigo has subsided. During, and often before, the paroxysms of vertigo the tinnitus may be more pronounced.

A peculiarity of the hearing loss associated with Ménière's disease is that in contrast to other types of perceptive impairment it is the low rather than the high tones that are the first to be involved. Between attacks the hearing may improve, although the extent of recovery tends to be less after each paroxysm. Some distortion, particularly in speech and musical sounds, may be experienced. There is also increased sensitivity to loud noises.

Ménière's disease usually begins between the ages of 30 and 50. Fortunately, in the majority of cases, only one ear is affected; in about 20 per cent both are affected. During the remission intervals most people can continue with their normal occupations and activities, and driving a car is not necessarily precluded. Working on ladders or at heights should, however, be avoided.

Another somewhat intimidating name for Ménière's disease is 'endolymphatic hydrops'; we now know that the symptoms are caused by a surplus of endolymphatic fluid in the inner ear. This surplus apparently increases the pressure in the scala media, causing a deterioration in the hair cells. At the same time the pressure overstimulates the semicircular canals on which depends our sense of balance, thereby producing the sensation of vertigo. The cause of the increased endolymphatic pressure has not been conclusively established.

Accurate diagnosis is essential since vertigo is not confined to Ménière's disease. Other ear conditions in which dizziness is a symptom may be harder to treat. The intervals between attacks make it difficult for an otologist to be sure whether an apparent improvement is due to his treatment or to natural causes.

Presbyacusis

Some degree of hearing loss is one of the burdens of old age. Of course not all old people are sufficiently hard of hearing to have difficulty in social situations. In every decade of life after 20, however, there is an increase in the proportion of us who are conscious of some deterioration in the acuity of our hearing. It has been estimated that about 25 per cent of 65-year-olds have more difficulty in hearing than they did at 30. At 70 and 80, the percentages increase to $33\frac{1}{3}$ and 50 per cent respectively.

Presbyacusis or 'senile deafness' is characterized by an increasing loss in the higher-frequency range. It becomes difficult to hear speech clearly; an old person will complain that people 'won't speak up'. When they do, recruitment or increased sensitivity to sound will lead to the complaint that 'there's no need to shout'. Recruitment also intensifies the difficulty of hearing in group situations where there is background noise.

There are various reasons why our hearing deteriorates in later life. Békésy points out that 'the ageing of the ear is not difficult to understand if we assume that the elasticity of the tissues in the inner ear declines in the same way as that of the skin: it is well known that the skin becomes less resilient as we grow old—a phenomenon anyone can test by lifting the skin on the back of his hand and measuring the time it takes to fall back.' This degeneration begins at the basal end of the cochlea and is accompanied by atrophic changes in the auditory nerve fibres.

An interesting problem, however, is why presbyacusis is more pronounced in certain people. The rate of degeneration may be influenced by the lifetime experience of the ear, particularly by its exposure to noise. A study by Rosen of the Maabaans, a primitive African tribe living in an environment where the noise level only occasionally exceeded 40db, indicated that a male Maabaan aged between 70 and 79 had keener hearing than a sample of Americans in the 30–39 age range who had been exposed to the noises of modern civilization (S. Rosen and others, 'Presbyacusis Study of a Relatively Noise-free Population in the Sudan', *Annals Otolaryngology and Rhinology*). An alternative hypothesis is that the absence of stressful living rather than merely of noise could be an important factor. One reason why women suffer less than men from hearing loss in age may be that they are less often exposed to noisy conditions at work. It is known that blood pressure and local atherosclerosis (hardening and thickening of the small arteries) may be connected with a limited hearing loss. Rosen has also attempted to show that a diet with a high fat content may lead not only to cardiovascular disease but to inferior hearing in later life. The apparent difference in the hearing ability of individuals of a given age may even be due to psychological factors. The author recalls reading about an old gentleman who after listening to a garrulous wife for almost fifty years had heard enough, and was happy to withdraw into the quiet world provided by impaired hearing.

TINNITUS

Tinnitus, the Latin word for 'ringing' or 'jingling' may be defined as a subjective experience of noise when there is no external stimulation. Head noises accompany almost all forms of hearing impairment and manifest themselves in a wide variety of ways. A somewhat pedantic distinction is occasionally made between tinnitus and 'auditory hallucination'. In tinnitus, the sounds heard are simple monotones, variously described as 'buzzing', 'ringing', 'throbbing' etc. In auditory hallucination, more complex and cacophonous sounds are experienced, so that the person concerned may complain of 'guns going off in his head' or 'a devil's orchestra'. One particularly unfortunate lady stated that her tinnitus sounded like 'the first three bars of God Save the Queen endlessly repeated'. Many people find their tinnitus more distressing than the loss of hearing.

The origins of tinnitus are as diverse as those of hearing impairment and possibly even more numerous. Three common causes are obstructions to sound conduction, pathological alterations in the cells of the cochlear sensory system and the physical distortion of the cochlear sensory system. Obstructions to sound conduction arise in the outer or middle ears and the resultant tinnitus can be due to wax, otitis-media or otosclerosis. Pathological changes can be brought about by noise and drugs.

Physical distortion of the cochlear system is usually responsible for the tinnitus that accompanies Ménière's disease.

Tinnitus may be confined to one ear, when it is indicative of a local cause, or be bilateral, which is symptomatic of a general condition. There is also a third type, central tinnitus, when the noises seem to be diffused all over the head rather than located specifically. Only rarely is central tinnitus due to an ear condition.

Tinnitus due to obstructions to sound conduction often disappears when the impediment is removed. One of the bonuses received by people who undergo successful surgery for otosclerosis can be the loss of their tinnitus, in addition to having their hearing restored to a serviceable level. In most cases, however, tinnitus is intractable. Sadly the only advice that the otologist can give is that the afflicted person must 'learn to live with his head noises'. Given courage and a constructive attitude it is possible to become at least partially accustomed to tinnitus. Some advice from a person who has lived with tinnitus for over forty years, Mr. C. H. Mardell, the present Secretary of the British Association of the Hard of Hearing, is useful:

> The best way to treat tinnitus is the same as one treats the club bore. You accept you must listen to him and you do so with the best grace you can. So if the head noises are unduly loud, to listen to them makes them acceptable as much as anything can; and trying to put them out of one's mind, being impossible, is a useless waste of emotion. This practice of listening to them does work and I would commend it as the only thing one can do to help, ie after a short while your mind wanders off them.

It is, of course, possible for your doctor to prescribe a mild sedative. Before asking him to do so, however, it is worth considering whether it is desirable to start a habit that might have to be continued for life. People often find that a more constructive approach is to keep the mind occupied by some absorbing hobby and to get as much healthy exercise as possible. Some tinnitus sufferers find temporary relief by blotting out the noises by turning up their hearing aids to secure maximum amplification. Some 30 per cent of persons afflicted by tinnitus may be assisted by a 'tinnitus masker'. This device, by feeding a band of white noise to the affected ear, has the effect of making the tinnitus either unaudible or less troublesome. Details of the tinnitus masker can be obtained from the RNID.

4 Measuring Hearing and Hearing Loss

Sound is one of the most important factors in our environment. In the form of speech, it is the most convenient form of communication. It is often a source of pleasure, as when we listen to music. When sound becomes excessive, distracting or even painful, such as the din of machinery in a factory, the blare of an unwanted radio or the scream of a jet engine we have the problem of noise. Without sound our world seems empty and dead.

If we know something of the nature of sound and its relationship to hearing, we can understand how our hearing may be measured and how such measurements can be used by an otologist to determine the nature of his patient's loss—and then what assistance he can provide.

SOUND AND DECIBELS

The sensation of hearing takes place when a stimulus called a 'sound' is detected by the ear. The source of this stimulus can always be traced to the movement or vibration of a body, although this movement may be so minimal or rapid that it cannot be seen. Place your fingers on your throat as you talk or sing and you will be able to feel your windpipe vibrating. Strike a tuning fork on the table and listen for its sound. If you then grasp the prongs you will feel the quivering metal.

Sound reaches the ear in the form of waves that originate at the sound source and travel through the air at about 344 metres per second. A sound wave is characterized by a to-and-fro movement known as compression and expansion. A vibrating body is surrounded by particles of air; as it vibrates the particles are first compressed or pushed outwards so that they collide with neighbouring particles. A chain reaction is thus set up—much as railway wagons push each other forward in a shunting operation. In between the movements the particles spread out again and expansion takes place. When a compression arrives at the ear, the slightly higher pressure causes the ear-drum to be pushed inwards; with expansion the pressure behind the drum causes it to bulge outwards.

Sound waves differ according to their complexity but with what is known as a pure-tone a sound wave may be pictured as in Fig 3.

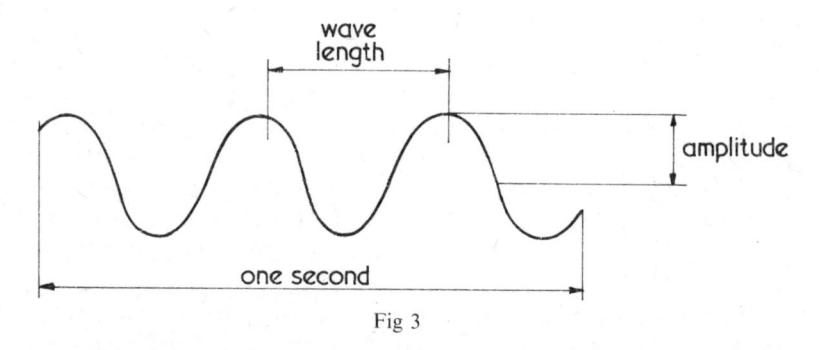

Fig 3

From the standpoint of this book the most important attributes of a sound wave are its frequency, pitch and intensity.

The *frequency* of a sound wave is the number of cycles of compression and expansion that take place within one second. The term 'cycles per second' has now been replaced by the expression Hertz (Hz). If, in one second, a sound results in 1,500 compressions and expansions it is said to have a frequency of 1,500 Hz. A young adult with normal hearing has an audible range from 15 Hz to about 20,000 Hz. Within this range the human ear is particularly sensitive to sounds that fall between 1,000 and 4,000 Hz. Sounds below the audible range are described as infrasonic while those above are referred to as ultrasonic.

The *pitch* of a sound is determined by the number of wave vibrations per second or Hz. The greater the length of a wave, the fewer will be the number of wavelengths passing a point in one second. Conversely the shorter the wavelength, the higher the pitch. A very low note, 15 Hz, has a wavelength of about 22 metres. A very high note, 20,000 Hz, has a wavelength of about 0.017 metres. As we grow older the sensitivity of our ears to high frequencies and the ability to hear high-pitched tones is progressively reduced.

Intensity is the amount of energy put into the sound by its source; this is shown by the amplitude of the sound wave. Loudness and intensity are different, but are related, since loudness depends on intensity. If we strike a tuning-fork gently, for example, it will produce a soft tone and will result in a wave of low amplitude. When the fork is struck more forcefully the tone will be louder and the amplitude of the wave will be greater. In both cases, however, the frequency of the note will be the same. As we know, sound fades as it travels through the air. As sound waves travel from their source, the amplitude of their compression-expansion is reduced as a function of the distance travelled. In simple terms this means that if you are in the open air listening to a person standing 2 feet away and he moves to a distance of 4 feet, his voice will sound not half but only one-quarter as loud as it did before. Every hearing-impaired person should therefore discover the approximate distance at which he can hear a conversation under different conditions, such as in a quiet room or out-of-doors, and ensure that he keeps within this range of the speaker.

Sound intensity can be measured in two ways, namely in terms of the *energy* given out by a source, eg the noise made by a jet aircraft taking off, or the variations caused in the normal atmospheric *pressure*. Sound energy and sound pressure are related. As can be seen from the table on page 30, sound energy increases as the square of sound pressure. Thus a tenfold increase in pressure corresponds with a hundredfold (10×10) increase in sound energy. For comparing changes in either energy or pressure we use *decibels*.

There are several reasons why decibels are confusing to people who are not physicists or mathematicians. Firstly, a decibel is not a unit such as a volt or metre, but a ratio. The noise produced by two bees will obviously be twice that of one bee. Similarly, if you listen to one jet aircraft and then to two planes simultaneously, the loudness will again be doubled. Although the noise of the jets will be vastly greater than the bees, the relative increase in sound will be the same in both cases. A given number of decibels therefore expresses the ratio of a measured amount of sound energy or sound pressure to a reference intensity or pressure. In a simplified form a decibel can be expressed as either

$$\frac{\text{sound energy}}{\text{reference sound energy}} \quad \text{or} \quad \frac{\text{sound pressure}}{\text{reference sound pressure}}$$

SOUND ENERGY AND SOUND PRESSURE UNITS AND THEIR DECIBEL EQUIVALENTS

RATIO EQUIVALENT SOUND ENERGY (POWER) RATIO	DECIBEL EQUIVALENT	SOUND PRESSURE RATIO
1:1	0	1:1
100:1	10	10:1 (10^1)
10,000:1	20	100:1 (10^2)
1,000,000:1	30	1,000:1 (10^3)
100,000,000:1	40	10,000:1 (10^4)
10,000,000,000:1	50	100,000:1 (10^5)
1,000,000,000,000:1	60	1,000,000:1 (10^6)
100,000,000,000,000:1	70	10,000,000:1 (10^7)

All measurements must start somewhere. If we measure the height of a mountain, for example, the reference point is sea level. With sound, the reference point is the threshold of hearing, which may be considered as the quietest pure tone audible at a given frequency to a person with normal hearing.

A second source of confusion is that we use different reference points in respect of sound energy and sound pressure. Where sound energy is concerned, power is measured in watts per square metre and the threshold of hearing is taken as 0.000,000,000,001 watts/m² or 10^{-12}/m² (ten to the minus twelve watt per square metre). Where sound pressure is used this is expressed in Newtons per square metre (N/m²) for which the term 'pascal' has been internationally agreed. One pascal is about ten-millionths of the normal atmospheric pressure. The threshold of hearing in this case is taken as 20 micro pascals or 0.00002 of a pascal. This latter reference was taken because it is the smallest sound pressure to which the ear will respond.

The table shows that the noise of a jet aircraft at 100 feet results in a sound pressure ratio 1,000,000 above the threshold of hearing, and a relative sound energy one billion (1,000,000×1,000,000) times greater than the softest sound detectable by a normal ear.

The table shows that the noise of a jet aircraft at 150 metres according to whether we are concerned with energy or pressure. For most of the applications in this book we are concerned with sound pressure. An audiogram specified in decibels shows how many times greater than normal a sound pressure of a given

DECIBEL EQUIVALENT	RELATIVE INTENSITIES (approximate examples)
0	Threshold of hearing
20	Still day in the country away from traffic
40	Rustle of leaves in gentle breeze
60	Normal conversation at distance of one metre in quiet room
80	Traffic in busy street
100	Very noisy factory (may damage hearing)
120	Jet aircraft taking off at 150 metres
140	At 140 db a sound will not be observed as such. The sensitive parts of the ear will be shaken so violently that the sensation will be experienced as pain rather than sound

frequency must be before it is just detectable. An ear with a 60 db impairment, for example, requires 1,000 times as much sound pressure to hear what is perceived at the same frequency by a normal ear.

A third point of difficulty is that billions and millions are cumbersome numbers. There is, however, a way out. Any number can be expressed in terms of 10 to a given power; eg 1,000 is 10x10x10, or 10^3. Originally sound was measured in terms of *Bels*, a unit named after Alexander Graham Bell. One Bel was equal to a tenfold increase in sound energy. Similarly three Bels corresponded to 10^3. Using this notation the awkward number of 1,000,000,000,000 used in the table can be reduced to 12 Bels or twelve tenfold increases. The Bel, however, was too large a unit for electronic engineers who required greater precision, and in 1929 the *decibel* or one-tenth of a Bel was universally adopted. The ratio of the jet noise to the reference intensity is, therefore, 60 decibels and 120 decibels for sound energy and sound pressure respectively.

AUDIOMETERS AND AUDIOMETRY

The modern instrument for measuring hearing is the audiometer. These vary in sophistication, but all of them incorporate three essential features: a frequency selector; a hearing-level selector; and a receiver, which may either be an earphone or a bone-conduction vibrator. The frequency selector selects the frequency at which the ear is to be tested. All audiometers test in steps of one octave at frequencies of 125, 250, 500, 1,000, 2,000, 4,000 and 8,000 Hz while for clinical work half-octave frequencies of 750, 1,500, 3,000 and 6,000 Hz are also provided. The hearing-level selector presents each frequency at a defined output pressure level, usually from minus 10 db to 100 db, which on modern audiometers is calibrated to the standard laid down in 1964 by the International Standards Organization. This standard set 0 db as the threshold of hearing for pure-tone audiometers, and was based on a survey of the hearing of a large number of otologically normal people aged 18–30 years. An 'otologically normal subject' was defined as 'a person in a normal state of health who is free from all signs or symptoms of ear disease and from wax in the ear canal and has no history of undue exposure to noise'. On most audiometers the hearing-level selector is divided into steps of 5 db.

In addition, audiometers are fitted with an interrupter switch, a masking device and a speech circuit. The interrupter switch is used to present or to withdraw a signal to the ear. The masking device is used when someone's two ears are markedly dissimilar in sensitivity: if the sound pressure required for audibility in the poorer ear is so high that the better ear picks up the signal, indirectly or by bone conduction, the accuracy of the test will be affected. Audiometers can present white noise or some other masking sound to the ear that is not being tested. (White noise is a continuous noise, eg the hissing of steam, in which high, middle and low frequencies are equally represented. As the power is distributed uniformly over the whole spectrum it is, by analogy with light, called white noise.) Like the hearing-level selector the masking dial, or noise attenuator as it is technically called, is usually in steps of 5 db.

For social adequacy the ability to hear speech is clearly more important than to detect pure tones. On audiometers designed to test both pure tones and speech, the speech circuit provides a means by which lists of words, either on pre-recorded tapes or spoken by the examiner, can be presented through the headphones or bone-conduction receiver. Speech audiometry is referred to in more detail below.

With a Békésy audiometer a person can administer his own hearing test. This machine is increasing in popularity because with it the pure tone threshold can be determined not only for the octave and half-octave frequencies but also for all the intermediate frequencies. Both standard and Békésy tests are recorded on a chart called an *audiogram* which shows the thresholds of hearing for a person at given frequencies. An example of a pure-tone audiogram is shown in Fig 4. The importance of the skill of the person administering the test cannot be overstressed.

The audiometer is a tool and as such it can be operated skilfully by the craftsman or clumsily and ineffectively by the amateur. The results of a hearing test must always be evaluated in terms of the individual who performs the test ... the audiogram is not a photograph of an individual's hearing loss; it is the best estimate by the audiometrist of the state of the patient's hearing based on his observation of the patient's behaviour in the testing situation (H. A. Newby, *Audiology*).

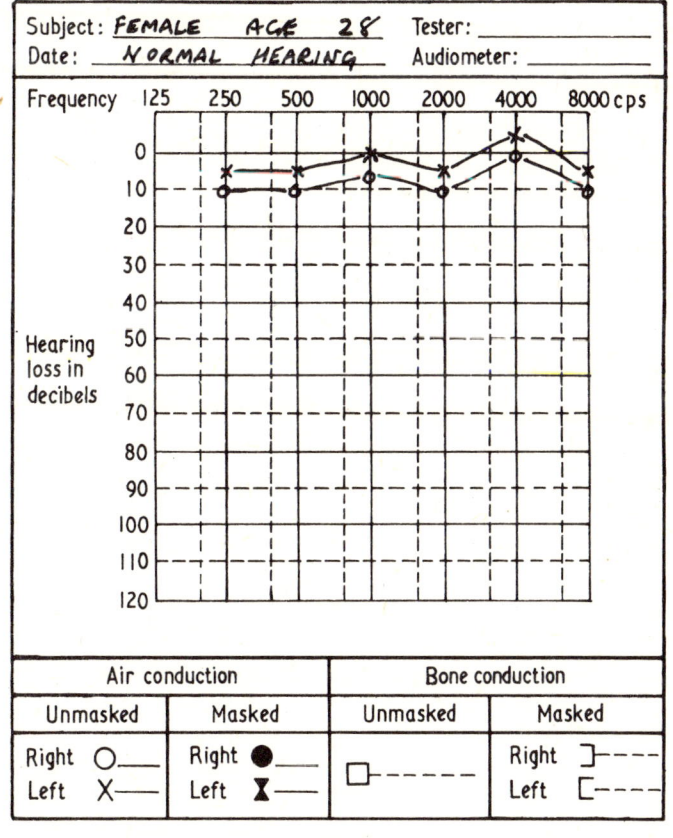

Fig 4

TAKING AN AUDIOMETRIC TEST

A routine audiometric test will usually consist of tests of your ability to hear pure tones by air and bone conduction, and to hear and understand speech. The tests required in your particular case will be specified by the otologist.

Pure Tone Testing

The object of pure-tone audiometry is to determine your threshold of hearing at selected frequencies. Pure tones are tested very simply. The tester will try the right ear first, except that if there is a marked difference in sensitivity he will start with the better ear. You indicate that you have heard the signal, by pressing a button which illuminates a bulb on the audiometer or by tapping the table, raising your finger or simply saying 'yes'. For air conduction, the tester will then place a pair of headphones on your head and ask you to face away from the audiometer.

It is usual for the tester to begin by establishing your hearing threshold at 1,000 Hz. There are two approaches to finding the threshold. In what is known as the *descending* method the tester will present a tone which, on the basis of his observations and information so far, he assumes you will be able to hear. Thus, at 1,000 Hz the hearing selector may be turned to 40 db. If you hear this tone the tester will turn it off with interrupter switch and turn the selector down by 10 db intervals until you are no longer able to hear the signal. The selector will then be turned up in 5 db steps until the signal is again heard. Once again the selector will be turned down in 5 db intervals until the sound is inaudible. This increasing and decreasing will be continued until you have made three consistent responses. The level of these responses will be taken as your threshold at 1,000 Hz.

The *ascending* method is broadly similar, except that, initially, the hearing selector will be set at −10 db and will be turned up in 5 db steps until you indicate that you are receiving the signal. Again your responses will be checked until you report three consistent indications of the threshold. After testing at 1,000 Hz other frequencies will be taken, usually beginning with the higher levels, ie 2,000, 4,000, 6,000, 8,000, and then reverting to the lower frequencies. The tester will plot your responses for each ear on the audiogram. As can be seen from Fig 3 the symbols O and X are used to indicate an air-conduction test for the right and left ears respectively. A red pen or pencil is often used to indicate bone conduction and blue for air conduction.

After the air-conduction tests have been completed the headphones will be taken off and a bone-conduction vibrator applied to the mastoid of one ear, unless there is a substantial difference between left and right when both ears, using masking, will be tested. The purpose of the bone-conduction test is to measure the sensitivity of the inner ear and the auditory nerve. By comparing your air and bone conduction thresholds, the otologist will be able to determine just where your hearing is impaired. If, for example, your bone conduction is normal but your air conduction is not, the trouble may be assumed to be some form of conductive impairment arising in either the outer or the middle ear. The threshold for bone conduction can never be lower than that for air conduction. With bone conduction a masking sound is usually presented to the opposite ear to ensure that the pure tone will only be perceived in the ear being tested.

Speech Testing

Helen Keller declared that 'the sound of the human voice is the most vital stimulus of all' because, as she says, 'it brings language, sets thoughts astir and keeps us in the intellectual company of man'. To discover what practical handicap for understanding speech results from the hearing disability, and the extent to which residual hearing can be used for everyday communication, it is necessary to supplement the information obtained from pure-tone tests by speech audiometry.

The procedures for speech audiometry are not very dissimilar to those for pure-tone testing. They basically consist of varying the intensity at which word or sentence lists are presented to each ear in turn, either by pre-recorded tapes or the live voice. The results of these tests are charted on a speech audiogram. One technique that differs from the pure-tone procedures is free-field testing, when the words are delivered at a measured level of loudness by a loudspeaker rather than through head-phones. Free-field testing is especially useful in helping to gauge the likely benefit of a hearing aid in normal circumstances.

The most important information obtained from speech audiometry is concerned with: your Speech Reception Threshold or SRT; your Speech Discrimination Score or PB; your Most Comfortable Loudness Level or MCL; your Threshold of Discomfort or TD.

The SRT is the lowest decibel level at which you can correctly score 50 per cent of a list of either monosyllabic or spondee words. (A 'spondee' is a word of two syllables in which equal stress is laid on each syllable, eg birthday, headlight.) This level approximates closely to the average of your thresholds for frequencies of 500, 1,000 and 2,000 Hz. As with pure-tone audiometry, your Speech Reception Threshold represents a comparison of your hearing for speech with the SRT of people with 'normal' hearing.

'Speech Discrimination' tests are even more helpful in measuring socially useful hearing. They are also of great value in distinguishing between conductive and sensorineural losses and in the prescription of suitable hearing aids. The words we use in speech are made up from speech sounds. These speech sounds consist of either consonants or vowels, and in English 16 vowel and 22 consonant sounds can be identified. Vowel sounds are easier to hear because they are lower in frequency and higher in intensity than consonants. Between the loudest vowel sound 'aw' and the softest consonant sound 'th' there is a difference of almost 30 db. In testing for intelligibility it would be ideal to use isolated speech sounds, but unfortunately these cannot be produced without considerable distortion. So the tester uses either lists of monosyllabic words, or short sentences in which the speech sounds occur with the same relative frequency as they do in ordinary spoken English. Such lists are called 'phonetically balanced' or PB lists. While, in principle, sentence tests are closer to the speech we all try to hear in everyday life, it has been found that in practice there is a close correlation between tests using sentences and single-word tests. Single-word tests are therefore used for speed and convenience, and sentence tests are valuable for people with a severe hearing loss who cannot understand speech at all without considerable help from the context.

In Britain, sentence and word articulation tests developed by D. B. Fry, Professor of Experimental Phonetics in the University of London, have been widely used. The sentence tests consisted of ten lists each of 25 sentences. The word-articulation tests had ten lists, each with 35 words of which 30 were of the consonant-vowel-consonant type and 5 either consonant-vowel or vowel-consonant. Recently much shorter lists of 10 words have been compiled by Arthur Boothroyd of the University of Manchester. The main distinction between the Fry and Boothroyd lists, apart from their length, is that the Boothroyd tests are scored on the basis of the number of speech sounds, rather than the number of words, correct. With word tests it has been found that normal conversation can be carried on at the decibel level at which a 50 per cent discrimination score is achieved.

The 'Most Comfortable Loudness' test indicates for each ear, or for both ears together when obtained by free-field testing, the number of db above the reference Speech Reception Threshold at which you can most easily understand speech. For people with normal hearing this will be about 40 db above their SRT. The normal SRT is 10 to 20 db above the normal pure-tone threshold at 500, 1,000 and 2,000 Hz.

As the term implies, your 'Threshold of Discomfort' is the number of db above zero SRT at which speech becomes uncomfortably loud or even painful. By subtracting your SRT from your Threshold of Discomfort the tester can ascertain your *dynamic range*. This indicates the range of useful hearing you have in each ear, and for both ears when a free-field test is given.

These speech tests obviously provide information that is vital both for diagnosing and for helping to overcome a hearing difficulty. Someone with an uncomplicated conductive impairment will understand speech if the sound is made loud enough. With sensorineural impairment, however, sound may result in yet further reduced intelligibility, due to what is known as *recruitment*. Recruitment is an exaggerated sensation of hearing following a slight increase in the intensity of sound. In an ear in which recruitment is absent, the 'Most Comfortable Loudness' level will be about 40 db above the Speech Reception Threshold. When recruitment is present the MCL may be only 10 db above the Speech Reception Threshold and, where it is marked, an increase of 15–20 db above the SRT may cause discomfort. Clearly this factor is of considerable importance when considering whether a hearing aid will help you.

THE MEASUREMENT OF HEARING HANDICAP

The results of audiometric tests provide the basis for an assessment of the degree of handicap experienced by a given person at a given time. For practical purposes it is often necessary to equate the quantitative measurement of hearing impairment shown by pure-tone audiogram with a given degree of disability. Such 'practical purposes' include compensation for industrial injury and decisions regarding an individual's suitability for special education, employment or military service. Decisions of this nature must also take other factors into account such as speech discrimination, the likely course of the impairment, the presence of tinnitus and vertigo and whether one or both ears are affected.

The first essential in deciding how much handicap a measured hearing impairment will cause is to decide the amount of loss that will constitute a given degree of disability. One such classification (formulated by the Committee on Conservation of Hearing of the American Academy of Ophthalmology & Otolaryngology) is shown in the table (page 39). The categories are based on the performance of the better ear at the three speech frequencies of 500, 1,000 and 2,000 Hz.

A second classification, by S. R. Mawson, a British otologist, is shown in the table at the top of opposite page.

One difficulty with such classifications is the lack of a recognized name to give the various categories of handicap. There is also some discrepancy between the degrees of loss considered appropriate to a particular category. A very crude relationship between hearing loss and difficulty in social situations is as follows:

HEARING LOSS	HANDICAP
0–25 db	Little difficulty in normal situations
25–40 db	Impairment for church or theatre
40–50 db	Difficulty in direct conversation
55+	Difficulty with the telephone
90+	Total deafness for speech

Clearly these estimates of the difficulty caused will be influenced by many factors, including the noise in the environment, the acoustics of a building and the extent to which speech discrimination has been affected by a particular ear condition.

INTERPRETING AUDIOGRAMS

The interpretation of audiograms is the province of the otologist and there are two reasons why it is dangerous for the layman to venture into this field. Firstly, an audiometric configuration may be the result of more than one cause; it is also necessary to consider the pure-tone audiogram together with a

CLINICAL CLASSIFICATION OF DEAFNESS

CLASSIFICATION	SOCIAL DIFFICULTY	CLINIC VOICE TEST	PURE TONE AUDIOGRAM
Normal Hearing	none	18 ft or more	no loss over 10 db
Slight Deafness	long-distance speech	not over 12 ft	10–30 db loss
Moderate Deafness	short-distance speech	not over 3 ft	up to 60 db loss
Severe Deafness	all unamplified voices	raised voice at meatus	over 60 db loss
Total Deafness	voices never heard	nil	over 90 db loss

Source: S. R. Mawson, *Diseases of the Ear* (by permission of the author).

CLASSES OF HEARING HANDICAP

HEARING THRESHOLD LEVEL (ISO)	CLASS	DEGREE OF HANDICAP	AVERAGE HEARING THRESHOLD LEVEL FOR 500, 1,000 AND 2,000 Hz IN BETTER EAR — more than	AVERAGE HEARING THRESHOLD LEVEL FOR 500, 1,000 AND 2,000 Hz IN BETTER EAR — not more than	ABILITY TO UNDERSTAND SPEECH
25	A	not significant		25 db (ISO)	no significant difficulty with faint speech
40	B	slight handicap	25 db (ISO)	40 db	difficulty only with faint speech
55	C	mild handicap	40 db	55 db	frequent difficulty with normal speech
70	D	marked handicap	55 db	70 db	frequent difficulty with loud speech
90	E	severe handicap	70 db	90 db	can understand only shouted or amplified speech
	F	extreme handicap	90 db		usually cannot understand even amplified speech

patient's case history and the signs and symptoms observed at the physical examination of his ears, nose and throat. Supplementary information will be obtained when necessary from speech and impedance audiometry. Secondly, the audiogram of an individual does not always correspond to a 'typical' pattern for a particular type of impairment.

Conductive impairments

Fig 5 is the pure-tone audiogram of a man with a conductive impairment due to otosclerosis in the right ear. It will be seen that at the time of the test the left ear was normal for all practical purposes. The bone-conduction curve for the right ear shows a characteristic pattern called the 'Carhart Notch'. An American otologist, Raymond Carhart, in 1951 reported that prior to surgery, at that time the fenestration operation, the bone conduction of people with otosclerosis could not be measured precisely because of an 'inner-ear conductive block' caused by the fixed stapes impeding the movement of the inner-ear fluids. On average this impedance resulted in a lowering of the bone-conduction threshold of 5 db at 500 Hz, 10 db at 1,000 Hz, 15 db at 2,000 Hz and 20 db at 4,000 Hz. It will be seen that on this audiogram the average losses reported by Carhart have been exceeded.

The difference between the bone and air conduction thresholds is the 'bone-air gap' and is a good indication of conductive impairment. If middle-ear surgery is recommended for the restoration of hearing, its principal aim is the reduction or elimination of this gap. Most conductive audiograms show a 'flat' curve for the air-conduction losses, with the greater losses occurring in the lower frequencies. While in this audiogram the flatness is not as pronounced as is often the case, the loss in the lower frequencies is clearly shown. By averaging the losses at frequencies of 500, 1,000 and 2,000 Hz, ie 70+65+50=62, we can estimate that the speech threshold in this case will be about 62 db.

Fig 6 is the speech audiogram of a case of otosclerosis with an average loss of from 50–55 db. On the left of the audiogram is the speech-discrimination curve for a person with normal hearing. It will be noticed that even someone with no impairment does not reach a discrimination score of 100 per cent until the intensity level is raised to about 55 db above the threshold. The discrimination curve of the person under test is parallel to that

[Audiogram chart]

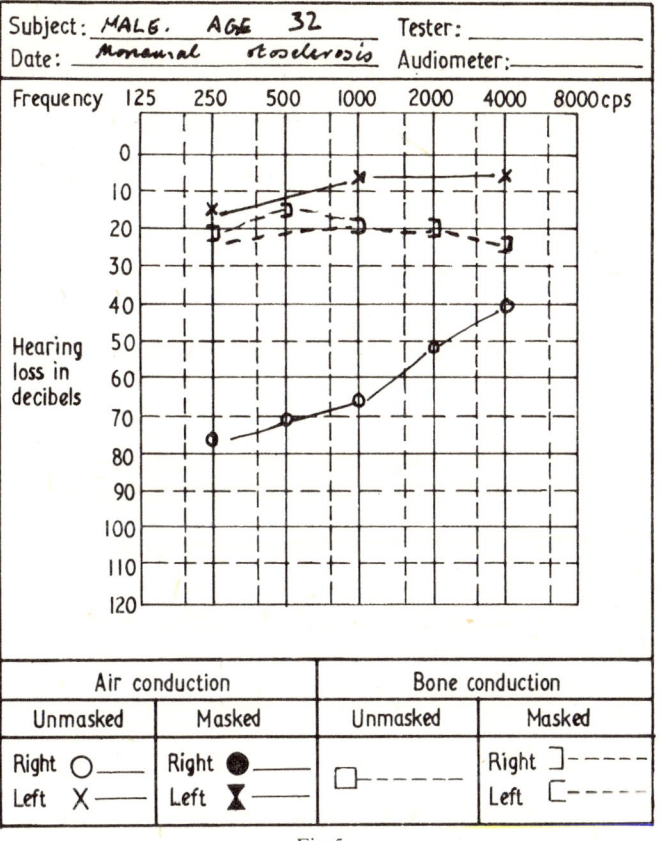

Subject: MALE. AGE 32   Tester: _____
Date: Monaural otosclerosis Audiometer: _____

Fig 5

for normal hearing. If the test words were presented more loudly, in this case at 80–90 db above the threshold, the otosclerotic will obtain the same score as the person with normal hearing. Thus, amplification by means of a hearing aid will enable the person with a pure conductive impairment to hear speech normally.

Sensorineural Impairments

Figs 7 and 8 show the pure-tone audiograms of two cases of sensorineural impairment. Fig 7 is the audiogram of a man aged 64 with presbyacusis, while Fig 8 refers to a woman aged 56 with Ménière's disease. In the former case it will be seen that the bone and air conduction thresholds are approximately equal, which is indicative of a sensorineural loss. In both instances there is near normal hearing at the lower frequencies with a fairly steep fall in

SPEECH TESTS
Material: ~~KT, NMP, MJ,~~ MJS, AB, ~~FRY~~   Method of scoring   Phonemes: ~~Words~~
Production: Tape: ~~Live voice~~   Presentation   Headphones: ~~Free field~~
Response   Spoken: ~~Written~~ : ~~Multiple choice~~

OTOSCLEROTIC   AV. LOSS
@ -55 d3.

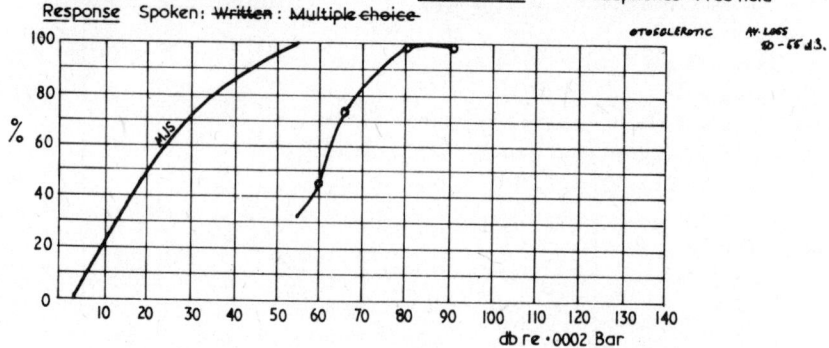

Fig 6

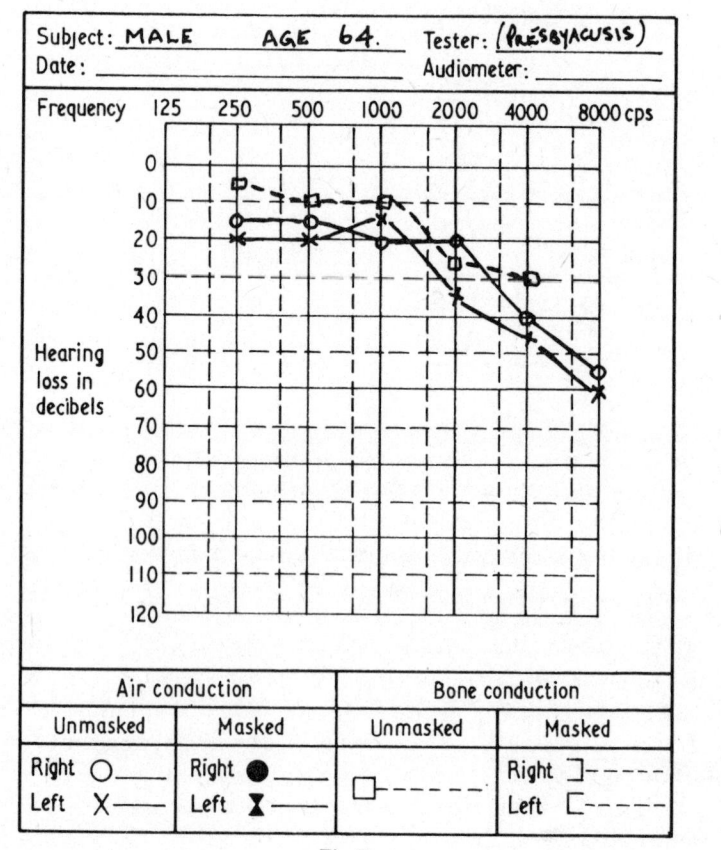

Subject: MALE   AGE 64.   Tester: (PRESBYACUSIS)
Date: Audiometer:

	Air conduction		Bone conduction	
	Unmasked	Masked	Unmasked	Masked
	Right ◯ ——	Right ● ——	◻ - - - - -	Right ⏋ - - - -
	Left ✕ ——	Left ⌛ ——		Left ⌐ - - - -

Fig 7

42

SPEECH TESTS
Material ~~KT, NMP, MJ, MJS~~, AB, ~~FRY~~   Method of scoring   Phonemes : ~~Words~~
Production : Tape : ~~Live voice~~   Presentation   Headphones : ~~Free field~~
Response   Spoken : ~~Written~~ : ~~Multiple choice~~

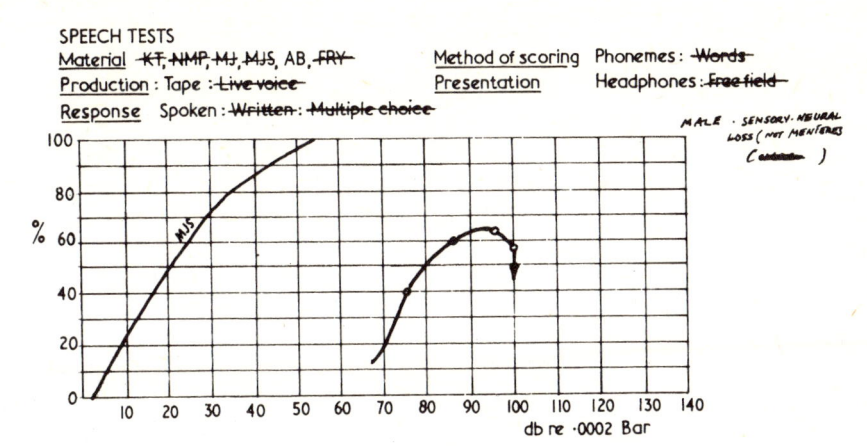

MALE : SENSORY-NEURAL
LOSS (NOT MENIERES)
( )

Fig 8

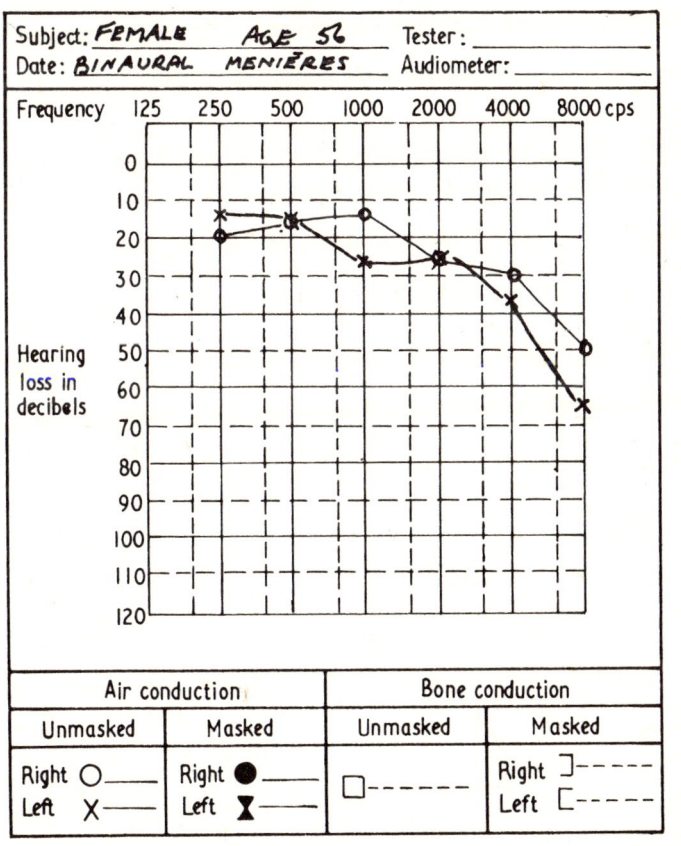

Subject: FEMALE   AGE 56   Tester: _____
Date: BINAURAL MENIÈRES   Audiometer: _____

Frequency 125 250 500 1000 2000 4000 8000 cps

Hearing loss in decibels

Air conduction		Bone conduction	
Unmasked	Masked	Unmasked	Masked
Right ○ —— Left X ——	Right ● —— Left ⊠ ——	□ ------	Right] - - - - Left [- - - -

Fig 9

the higher ranges. The practical effect is that while the lower-pitched vowel sounds will still be audible there will be difficulty in hearing the higher-pitched consonant sounds.

Fig 9 is the speech audiogram of a person with a sensorineural loss. Not until the intensity level is raised to 80 db above the threshold is he able to hear correctly 50 per cent of the words comprising the test. At 95 db his score improves to 65 per cent. After this point, however, discrimination deteriorates as amplification increases; thus, if the intensity level is raised to 100 db his score declines to 55 per cent. Parabolic curves are never found with pure conductive impairments; they do, however, illustrate the effect of recruitment, and how important it is to take this factor into account in the prescription of hearing aids.

5 You and Your Otologist

The most constructive advice that can be given to someone with any form of ear trouble is 'visit an otologist'. The person with a longstanding hearing impairment who has not seen an ear specialist during the last 15–20 years should also do so; he or she might possibly be helped by one of the developments that have taken place within this period. Even octogenarians have successfully undergone stapedectomy operations for the relief of otosclerosis. Accurate information on the type of loss and its cause is essential before a person with impaired hearing can be helped. Only an otologist can assemble this.

How does an ear specialist arrive at a diagnosis of what is wrong, and what steps might he take to cure or at least ameliorate the impairment?

VISITING THE OTOLOGIST

First ask your general practitioner to give you a letter of introduction to an ear specialist. If you feel you need advice on your ear trouble do not be dissuaded from your resolve. Not all doctors are interested in ears or keep abreast of progress in this field, and people with hearing impairments have sometimes been wrongly advised that nothing could be done for them. Syringing and eardrops will only relieve a loss of hearing due to wax in the outer ear.

Your doctor should know who is the best available specialist for you to see; the more knowledgeable he is about ears, the more information he will have about the reputations of otologists. There is nothing to stop you asking to be referred to a particular consultant. Your doctor may arrange for you to see an otologist without cost at the outpatients department of a hospital. Under the National Health Service, however, you have no automatic right to see a particular consultant at his outpatients clinic. You may, alternatively, prefer to see the consultant in his rooms, in which case a fee will be payable. While ultimately the diagnosis and treatment will be the same, I believe that it is more informative to see the otologist privately the first time. This does not imply any criticism of the National Health Service: it is simply based on the personal experience that in a busy hospital clinic the otologist has less time to explain the nature of your ear condition and to answer questions than in the quietness of his consulting rooms, where he is free from other distractions.

The consultant will be listed in either the Medical Directory or the Medical Register (available in most public reference libraries). He will almost certainly hold the Fellowship of one of the three Royal Colleges of Surgeons (London, Edinburgh or Dublin). The convention is that a surgeon is addressed as Mr, a physician as Dr.

THE OTOLOGIST'S DIAGNOSIS

Like a detective the otologist seeks his clues from three sources, the victim, the site of the crime and independent witnesses.

The first clues come from the victim—yourself. The otologist will want background details that only you can provide, so reflect on the following questions before you see him.

1. Which of the following symptoms are present: (a) a hearing loss; (b) head noises; (c) dizziness; (d) discharge from the ear; (e) earache?

2. For how long have I been troubled by these symptoms?

3. What events do I associate with the onset of my ear trouble—an accident, colds, noise, pregnancy, worry, etc?

4. Have any members of my family had impaired hearing?

5. Do I hear better in a noise?

6. Do I find loud noises or speech uncomfortable?

The helpfulness of your answers to such questions will be enhanced if you have given them some prior thought. For example, grandfather's 'deafness' which only became marked in his 80s was probably due to presbyacusis, and is not significant. Aunt Mary who 'went deaf' at 30 is worth reporting. It is also helpful to the consultant if you can explain in simple terms not merely that you have tinnitus, but whether it is intermittent or continuous and affects one or both ears. On his side, the consultant will have been noticing some of the signs mentioned in Chapter 3, such as whether you speak softly or loudly, strain to catch his speech or try to lip-read what he is saying.

The second set of clues will be obtained from an examination of your ears, nose and throat. The otologist will be particularly interested in your ear-drums and eustachian tubes. He will note whether the ear-drums are normal or if they are perforated; in otitis-media the drums may bulge outward or be drawn inwards. Changes in the colour and texture of the drums may also provide clues to what is wrong. Similarly the consultant will want to know whether your eustachian tubes are functioning efficiently. You may be asked to pinch your nostrils and puff out your cheeks so that the effect on your hearing and ear-drums can be checked. The otologist will also examine your nose and throat for abnormalities that may cause ear trouble or aggravate an existing condition.

The third set of clues will be obtained from audiometric or tuning-fork tests. Before audiometers, otologists had to rely on tuning forks to determine the upper and lower tone limits within the speech range, and distinguish between conductive and sensorineural impairments.

The three most important tuning-fork tests are known as Weber, Rinne and Schwabach after their originators. The Weber test is used to determine whether hearing impairment affecting only one ear is conductive or perceptive, by comparing the bone conduction of both ears. A vibrating tuning fork is placed in the middle of the forehead. The person under test is asked to state whether he hears the sound in his good or his impaired ear. If the sound is heard in the impaired ear the bone conduction must be better in this ear than the other and the trouble will be conductive. If the sound is heard better in the good ear the hearing loss in the opposite ear will be sensorineural.

The Rinne test depends on the fact that with normal hearing a tuning fork held close to the ear will be heard (by air conduction) for about twice as long as one placed on the mastoid (heard by bone conduction). A vibrating fork is therefore held just outside the ear passage. When the person under test no longer hears the vibrations the fork is transferred to the mastoid. Both ears are tested in this way. If the vibrations are heard longer by bone than by air conduction, that is evidence of a conductive impairment.

The Schwabach test compares the bone conduction of a

person with a hearing difficulty to that of someone assumed to have normal hearing. The vibrating tuning fork is placed on the mastoid of the patient. When he no longer hears the vibrations the fork is immediately transferred to the mastoid of the otologist. If the otologist continues to hear the vibrations it suggests that the patient has a sensorineural loss.

Although the Weber, Rinne and Schwabach tests are still used, most otologists now prefer to rely on the information obtained from audiometric tests, mainly because: such tests are quantitative and objective, rather than qualitative and subjective; audiograms show the pattern of hearing impairment by enabling typical configurations to be identified; audiograms can be kept by the otologist, and used to measure the extent of deterioration during a given period, or the extent of improvement obtained from treatment; audiograms can be used to prescribe the type of hearing aid most likely to benefit a given individual.

It must be stressed, however, that neither tuning-fork nor audiometric tests do anything more than provide evidence about the type of hearing impairment. The otologist can only form a reliable opinion on the degree of loss when, in addition to the tests, he has considered the clues provided by the hearing-impaired person himself and by the physical examination of the patient's ears, nose and throat.

WHAT CAN THE OTOLOGIST DO?

The otologist will seek to achieve one or more of the following objectives: the elimination of infection; the restoration or improvement of hearing; the relief of tinnitus and vertigo.

The Elimination of Infection

As explained in Chapter 3, most acute infections of the middle ear are due to bacteria spreading up the eustachian tube as a result of colds, tonsillitis and similar conditions. Before about 1938 acute otitis-media was attended by the very real danger that an infection of the middle ear might invade the mastoid process and, unless relieved by prompt surgery, result in such potentially fatal complications as meningitis or a brain abscess.

Many older people will recall at school contemporaries who 'had a mastoid' and ugly-looking scars behind the ear to prove it.

To prevent the accumulation of pus and the perforation of the ear-drum the usual procedure was *myringotomy*, the surgeon making an incision in the ear-drum for the double purpose of relieving pain and allowing the fluid to escape. Myringotomy is still occasionally performed when other procedures fail to give relief, especially when the eustachian tube is blocked with the result that the middle ear is inadequately ventilated. In the latter case the otologist may insert a small dumbbell-like tube or 'grommet' through the myringotomy to prevent the absorption by the middle ear's mucous membrane of the remaining air and its replacement by fluid. The grommet maintains atmospheric pressure in the middle ear, and when the drum is retracted the insertion of the tube usually leads to an improvement in hearing.

The dramatic fall in the incidence of mastoid infection and its complications since 1938 has been due to the effects of sulpha drugs and antibiotics. Their advent revolutionized otology, as it did most other branches of medicine. Far fewer myringotomies were needed, since antibiotics given early in otitis-media control the infection so that the condition resolves without rupture of the ear-drum. Even if a perforation has taken place the ear-drum heals with minimal scarring so that the hearing is not permanently impaired. The emergency mastoid operation ceased to be commonplace. Many ear conditions that had formerly required the attention of the specialist otologist could be treated as a matter of routine by the general practitioner. The knowledge that infection could be controlled gave otologists the confidence to develop modern surgical procedures for the ear.

There are, however, complications in the use of antibiotics. One such complication, the so called 'glue ear', has already been mentioned in the discussion of otitis-media in Chapter 3. Another danger is that the use of the antibiotic may be discontinued before it has completely eliminated the infection. When an antibiotic has been prematurely abandoned the re-emergence of resistant strains of bacteria is encouraged. It appears that the fire has been put out, but the underlying infection is smouldering, ready to flare up later in the form of 'masked mastoiditis' with its attendant dangers. The need for surgery for the removal or prevention of ear infections has not been entirely eliminated by the use of antibiotics. A familiar example is the removal of chronically affected adenoids that may be responsible for the infection or obstruction of the eustachian tube.

The Restoration or Improvement of Hearing

'There are two kinds of deafness. One is due to wax and curable, the other is not due to wax and is not curable.' So declared Sir William Wilde, FRCS, the father of Oscar Wilde. William Wilde, one of the first surgeons to take a special interest in otology, lived between 1815 and 1876, and until after World War II his statement was still substantially true except that, as we have seen, the incidence of hearing impairment had been significantly reduced by the use of antibiotics. Especially in the field of conductive impairment the situation has now changed dramatically, due to the development of the operating microscope, the control of infection by antibiotics and the work of a small group of pioneers who build on the foundations laid by earlier surgeons.

These three factors have led to two important developments in the field of middle-ear surgery. The first, tympanoplasty, attempts to deal with hearing impairment due to such conditions as injury to the drum and the effects of chronic otitis-media. The second, stapedectomy, is concerned with relieving hearing loss arising from otosclerosis.

Tympanoplasty. Tympanoplasty is the term for a group of procedures aimed at eradicating disease and restoring the sound-conducting mechanism of the middle ear. The procedures involved in tympanoplasty may be subdivided into myringoplasty and ossiculoplasty.

Myringoplasty seeks to repair the ear-drum where a perforation is too large to repair by other means. In effect the hole is 'patched' by tissue usually taken from the temporal muscle. Such repairs can, of course, be made only when the ear is free from discharge.

Ossiculoplasty is the reconstruction of the ossicular chain, the three small bones of the middle ear popularly termed the hammer, anvil and stirrup. These may become immobile or broken by disease or injury. Destructive disease in the middle ear, for instance, usually affects the anvil or incus, which being in the centre of the chain has the worst blood supply. The surgeon may place the patient's own incus in a new position; he may use an artificial replacement for a part of the chain; he may even use replacement ossicles removed from other people in the course of middle-ear operations. Some people actually bequeath their ossicles to be removed after their deaths and used in replacement surgery.

Since tympanoplasty was first described in 1953 much has been done to improve the results obtained. Not until the surgeon has inspected the middle ear through his operating microscope does he know precisely the repairs that are necessary to improve hearing. Tympanoplasty techniques therefore require great skill, patience and ingenuity from the otologist.

Stapedectomy. Surgical attempts to restore hearing lost through otosclerosis have taken three separate paths.

The first, *fenestration*, attempted to bypass the fixed stapes through the creation of a new window or fenestra in the labyrinth. This window enabled sound vibrations to be transmitted via the inner-ear fluids to the round window. The first attempt to create a new window was made in 1897, but the improvement in hearing resulting from early efforts was temporary, in most cases lasting for only a few days. It was not until about 1938 that a simplified one-stage operation was developed by Julius Lempert of New York, that really put fenestration on the otological map.

Some excellent results were obtained, but there were a number of disadvantages. Fenestration remained a major operation, requiring two to three weeks in hospital followed by a lengthy period of outpatient treatment. Often there were complications such as dizziness and discharge. Most seriously, hearing tended to deteriorate to the pre-operative level, due to the closure of the fenestra by a new overgrowth of spongy bone. This latter factor was frustrating to the otologist and distressing to the patient.

The second approach, that of *mobilisation of the stapes*, was used by early otologists, but their poor results and the high danger of serious infection in the pre-antibiotic era led to its abandonment until it was 'accidentally' rediscovered in 1952 by Samuel Rosen of New York. While preparing to perform a fenestration operation Rosen moved the patient's stapes just as a metal pan fell on the floor in an adjoining room. The patient remarked that he had heard something fall, whereupon Rosen whispered very softly, 'Do you like scrambled eggs?' 'Yes,' was the reply, 'and I heard every word.'

In a sense, stapes mobilisation was the direct opposite of fenestration. It was a much simpler operation requiring only a short stay in hospital and without post-operative complications. Sometimes near-normal hearing could be restored, a considerable advance on the best that could be expected from fenestration. Moreover, even if unsuccessful, stapes mobilisation did not prevent a fenestration operation later. It had its disadvantages, however. The stapes might become refixed by the pathological process of otosclerosis, and also there were dangers in the operation itself. Though for a time stapes mobilisation tended to be regarded as a 'nothing-to-it' operation, in which the stapes was given a little wiggle and hearing was miraculously restored, it soon emerged that great care was needed from the surgeon. If the stapes was moved a little too hard a loss of 60 db or more could occur, or it might even be pushed into the inner ear, resulting in no hearing at all.

The third and most successful approach, *stapedectomy*, involves the complete or partial removal of the stapes. Like fenestration and stapes mobilisation, it had been attempted by earlier otologists and abandoned because of the technical difficulties. It was not until 1956 that John Shea, jnr, of Tennessee performed the first stapedectomy involving the use of a prosthesis, an artificial part. In Shea's original operation the stapes was completely removed, the oval window thus being left open and its closure being effected by a graft consisting of a small segment of vein removed from the patient's arm. A polythene strut was then used to bridge the gap between the incus and the vein graft. In 1963 Shea started to use a piston made of Teflon, a plastic material, rather than a polythene strut. Subsequently other types of pistons have been devised, as have alternatives to vein graft for closing the oval window.

Stapedectomy is now the standard surgical procedure for the improvement of hearing impairment caused by otosclerosis. It does not cure the otosclerosis, but in the overwhelming majority of cases, it does give long-lasting serviceable hearing to people who little more than a quarter of a century ago could not have had much done for them.

As the operation will be of great interest and importance to many readers of this book, an attempt will be made to deal with some of the queries that must occur to anyone with otosclerosis. The answers given can be no more than generalisations, of course, and each individual must discuss his case with an otologist.

What are the main factors that the otologist considers in determining whether or not a person is suitable for stapedectomy surgery?

1 Correct diagnosis.

2 The state of the nerve of hearing, as shown by the extent to which pure tones are heard better by bone conduction than air conduction. The aim of the operation is, in fact, to close the gap between hearing by bone and by air conduction as shown by an audiogram. Ideally the loss by air conduction should be between 30 and 60 decibels.
3 Absence of infection.

Is stapedectomy precluded if I am over 60 years of age?

No.

Assuming that the otologist considers me suitable for stapedectomy, what in percentage terms are the chances of a substantial improvement in my hearing?

Better than 95 per cent.

Is there any danger that my hearing may be worse after a stapedectomy operation?

Yes. Sensorineural loss occurs in about 2 per cent of cases. It may occur at the time of the operation, or in about 1 per cent of cases some time afterwards.

What is the alternative to a stapedectomy?

The use of a hearing aid. There may be little point in encouraging an elderly person who has already become well adjusted to the use of a hearing aid to undergo stapedectomy. With younger people the abandonment of a hearing aid may be desirable for social and vocational reasons.

If I have a stapedectomy, for how long am I likely to be in hospital and away from work?

About a week in hospital and a further one to two weeks away from work.

Is the operation performed under a general or local anaesthetic?

Most surgeons operate with general anaesthesia. (I myself, however, had two stapedectomies performed under local anaesthesia and was comfortable throughout—more comfortable, in fact, than during many visits to the dentist.)

If the operation is successful will my hearing be restored immediately?

Sometimes there is an immediate hearing improvement that may temporarily disappear. Hearing usually returns in 2–4 weeks.

If one ear is successfully treated is it possible to perform a second stapedectomy on the other ear at a later date?

This question is debatable. Some otologists believe that because of the slight danger of late sensorineural loss it is undesirable to operate on both ears. (I had a stapedectomy on each ear and have a good result ten years later.) A middle-of-the-road view is that a period of at least five years should be allowed to elapse before an operation on the second ear is contemplated.

Is the hearing improvement likely to be permanent?

Yes, in the majority of cases. Among the causes of post-operative conductive loss are the slipping of the prosthesis and a leak of inner-ear fluid (perilymph) from the oval window.

If the hearing does regress after an initially successful stapedectomy, is it possible for the surgeon to rectify matters?

He has to decide whether or not to undertake a 'revision' operation. Where the loss is due to the slipping of the prosthesis the bone-air gap can be restored to within 10 db in about half of all cases.

Will a stapedectomy relieve or cure tinnitus?

Where the tinnitus is due to otosclerosis, and not to other causes, a successful stapedectomy will often cure it.

Vertigo and Tinnitus

Vertigo and tinnitus, which was discussed in Chapter 3, may be troublesome and even distressing accompaniments to hearing impairment. Vertigo can occur independently of conditions arising primarily in the ear. It may be due to such causes as high blood pressure, drugs and virus infections. A thorough medical examination is usually required to establish the reason for 'dizziness' or 'lightheadedness', and this examination will, if necessary, be supplemented by an otologic investigation.

While vertigo is not necessarily due to Ménière's disease, the treatment of this condition illustrates some of the approaches that have been made to the relief of dizziness arising from what is technically known as endolymphatic hypertension. These approaches may be classified in the order in which they are usually tried by the otologist, under the headings of diet, drugs and surgical intervention.

The dietary treatment is to restrict the intake of salt and fluid, in an attempt to reduce the excessive water pressure in the endolymphatic sac in the inner ear, which is a feature of Ménière's disease. Salt is important in this context since its consumption increases the amount of fluid in the body. In general, the diet will specify that salt should be eliminated from cooking and discontinued as a condiment. Bacon, breakfast cereals, cheese, ham, kippers, salt-butter and other foods with a high salt content should also be avoided. At the same time the daily intake of fluid should not exceed $2\frac{1}{2}$ pints (1.5 litres). The results of this regimen vary from person to person, and while many otologists commence treatment with a salt-controlled diet not all are convinced of its effectiveness.

When diet does not give relief the otologist may next prescribe drugs, particularly those that expand the arteries, the vasodilators. These drugs are used on the theory that the supply of the endolymph fluid may be affected by the blocking of the branch vessels of the internal auditory artery due to over-activity of the central nervous system. The function of vasodilators such as nicotinic acid is to dilate the auditory artery and its branches, with the object of restoring the blood supply and thus normalising the output of endolymph. Antihistamine drugs, popularly known by their proprietary names such as avomine and dramamine, are also prescribed, mainly because of their sedative effect.

The otologist will usually consider surgical intervention only when diet and drugs have failed to give relief. A number of operations have been devised aimed at the relief of vertigo in one of three ways; the control of endolymph production; the reduction of endolymph pressure; or the destruction of the vestibular labyrinth.

These procedures vary in complexity from the simple insertion of a grommet into the ear-drum to the selective destruction of the vestible by ultrasonic radiation. This last operation, first introduced in 1952, is usually advocated when only one ear is affected and there is serviceable hearing that the otologist is anxious to preserve.

6 Hearing Impairment is more than Dull Ears

Most people with normal hearing have little idea of the emotional and behavourial consequences of impaired hearing. An understanding of these consequences is important for at least two good reasons. Firstly, adjustment is often helped when a handicapped person knows something about what causes the feelings to which he may be prone. Secondly, a better understanding of the disability may assist his family and friends to give more constructive help.

EFFECTS ON FEELINGS AND BEHAVIOUR

A sudden loss of hearing is fortunately much less common than a gradual deterioration. A few people are, through disease or accident, faced with the traumatic experience of having to make a sudden transition from normal hearing to deafness. Far more often the loss of hearing is progressive, and the individual is able to adjust gradually to his limitations. Even in the early stages of progressive hearing loss, however, some behavioural characteristics may be seen. Although the person may not be regarded as 'deaf', his associates may notice that he is preoccupied, unsociable and absent-minded, and comment that 'he lives in a world of his own', is 'slow on the uptake' or 'hears only what he wants to hear'. If and when the loss becomes sufficiently severe to be a practical handicap, and especially when it cannot be remedied by surgical or other means, the person concerned is likely to experience both fear and depression.

The fear is usually due to uncertainty about the effect of the hearing loss on a way of life previously taken for granted. Family relationships, employment prospects, or even the capability to retain a job at all, may all be causing anxiety. The dulling of the asthetic pleasures of music, inability to enjoy convivial company, become haunting possibilities. Every social encounter holds the threat that by giving a wrong answer or behaving inappropriately he may appear stupid. Even a casual request for directions from a passing motorist may be a source of embarrassment.

Fear, however, tends to be an initial reaction to hearing loss and diminishes as one adjusts to the disability and learns how to cope successfully with some of the problems. Depression is more persistent. The causes of the depression are varied. As explained later in this chapter it may result from a sensation of 'deadness' often accompanied by a vague feeling of insecurity. The depression may also be accentuated by tinnitus or the influence of fatigue caused by the energy expended in trying to cope with the demands of an environment in which good hearing is taken for granted. This feeling of depression has been poignantly described by Jack Ashley, MP, who in 1967 became totally deaf as a result of a virus infection: 'I sat alone on the terrace [of the Houses of Parliament] watching the Thames. It looked bleak and cold. It was early evening and although I did not expect the river to be busy it seemed exceptionally still—and silent. I thought I had known despair, but now I felt a chill and deeper silence, as if a part of me was dead.'

The emotions of fear and depression may express themselves in outward conduct. An experiment conducted by an American psychologist, Lee Meyerson, provides some revealing insights into the ways in which loss of hearing may affect behaviour. He stopped the ears of some volunteers with cotton and wax plugs for a period of twenty-four hours. Their hearing loss was moderate, about 30 decibels—insufficient to prevent a tête-a-tête conversation but enough to cause difficulty in hearing speech in a large room. The volunteers were, of course, aware that their 'deafness' was only temporary and that with the removal of the plugs normal hearing would be restored at once. Yet within the short duration of the experiment, a number of characteristic responses to hearing loss were reported.

Some participants stated that they had tried to *withdraw* from social situations which were perceived as threatening: 'I was conscious of trying to remain aloof so that the girls at the table would ignore me. I felt as if I would like to go out of the house and be alone all day.' 'I pretended to be in a terrible hurry getting ready to leave so I wouldn't have to talk to anyone and maybe not understand what they had said.'

Other volunteers mentioned *aggressive* reactions. One who had experienced difficulty in following a lecture observed: 'The instructor talked in a very low voice. I spent most of the time thinking about how poor a teacher he was, how emotionally maladjusted he must be and calling him every name I could think of.' Sometimes the feelings of aggression were vented on others: 'My wife asked me why I had been so irritable and nasty all day.' Reference was also made to paranoid reactions such as *suspiciousness*: 'I knew they probably weren't but I couldn't help feeling that maybe they were talking about me.'

Attempts to conceal the supposed impairment by *bluffing* were reported: 'When they smiled, I smiled. When they laughed, I laughed: the rest of the time I made myself as inconspicuous as possible and prayed for the evening to come to an end.' Some comments revealed that inadequate hearing had resulted in *inappropriate behaviour*: 'Once I thought the situation was humorous and could not resist a grin. Jane explained later that the girl was very ill and seeking advice whether to go to hospital.'

Two other experiences reported were those of *embarrassment* arising from misunderstanding conversation and *lack of self-confidence* in associating with people that had developed into a diffused feeling of uneasiness and restlessness.

The reactions are typical of those experienced by hearing-impaired people in real-life situations. Also, a conclusion reached by Meyerson is worth quoting verbatim: 'The psychologically and socially undesirable behaviour that has been reported for physically handicapped persons does not arise because the disabled are different kinds of people but because they have been subjected to different kinds of life experiences.'

WHY THESE EFFECTS OCCUR

Three possible reasons why impaired hearing may have these effects are: loss of 'affective tone', frustration, and social attitudes to disability.

Loss of Background Noise

An interesting theory about the cause of the depression that often accompanies impaired hearing has been put forward (by D. A. Ramsdell in Hallowell Davis, *Hearing and Deafness*). He states that sound is normally perceived simultaneously at three levels, 'primitive', 'warning' and 'symbolic'. The primitive level is the constantly changing pattern of background noise to which we give no attention unless our interest is consciously aroused. Thus, it is only when I stop writing this page and consciously *listen* that I become aware that a bird is singing outside my window, the television is on in another room and a car is passing the house. When we actively respond to auditory signals, as for example footballers to a referee's whistle, we are hearing at the warning level. The most complex level of hearing is the use of sounds as symbols for the purpose of communication, as when we transmit and receive messages in the course of conversation. Ramsdell believes that it is the diminution or loss of hearing at the primitive, rather than the symbolic, level that is responsible for the depressive effects of impaired hearing.

The loss of the sensation of background noise has a twofold effect. Firstly, it is this background noise, or 'affective tone' as it is termed, that makes each of us feel that we belong to our environment. When this tone is lost there is a profound feeling of solitariness and social isolation. One has only to consider how much the enjoyment of a football match is heightened by the 'atmosphere' generated by the roaring and singing of the crowd. Secondly, hearing at the primitive level increases both our sense of security in the present and our ability to cope with future situations. Hearing can warn us of dangers that we cannot see. We may hear footsteps approaching in the dark even though we cannot see the walker. When crossing the road we cannot look in two directions at the same time but, looking left, we can rely on our hearing to warn of traffic coming from the right. Without this auditory alertness it is not surprising that a hearing-impaired person feels insecure and uncertain in his environment. Such feelings are strong contributory factors to depression.

Frustration

Frustration arises from the hearing-impairment barrier which prevents the attainment of many desirable goals. I may, for example, wish to listen to a lecture given by a famous authority on a subject in which I am interested, but I am frustrated because I cannot hear what he has to say. Nor can I keep pace with office or family conversations.

Reactions to frustration may be either positive or negative. Positive reactions include problem solving, accepting substitute goals and finding a compensation. One common negative response is that of aggression, which can take three main forms.

It can be physical, as when a direct attack is made on the barrier that causes the frustration. Aggression may, of course, also be positive—as when, through a surgeon, we attack the bony growth that prevents the movement of the stapes in otosclerosis. Aggression may be verbal, when we relieve pent-up frustration by cursing the loss of hearing that prevents the attainment of so many goals. There is also substitute aggression in which a person vents all his tension on his family and friends. It will be recalled that one of Meyerson's volunteers reported 'my wife asked me why I had been so irritable and nasty all day'. An understanding of the causes of this substitute aggression may make it easier to live with a hearing-impaired person and improve the quality of his personal relationships.

Other negative reactions which may afflict a person with a loss of hearing are those of regression, fixation, withdrawal and resignation. We regress when we engage in childish forms of behaviour such as weeping or temper tantrums. Fixation is a compulsion to continue with a type of behaviour that will accomplish nothing towards the removal of the frustrating barrier. Sadly, people who have been advised by a competent otologist that nothing can be done to cure the hearing loss will often continue to visit other ear specialists in the vain hope that one will have some remedy unknown to the others. Worse still, they go to quacks and charlatans who have no qualms about prescribing useless and expensive appliances or courses of treatment. Withdrawal has already been noted as a response which may be adopted by a person who finds that interaction with the hearing world imposes too great a strain. Resignation may be the end result of prolonged frustration; the individual no longer seeks constructive ways of dealing with his disability and gives up, lapsing eventually into apathy and despair.

Social Attitudes

The attitudes of a person with impaired hearing are only partially derived from the actual handicap. They are also affected by the social attitudes shown by non-handicapped people. A disabled person may come to accept the attitudes he has encountered from society as his own.

Two sociological terms that help us to understand social attitudes to hearing impairment are 'deviance' and 'stigma'. Deviant behaviour violates the generally accepted norms of society. It is generally assumed that we live in a hearing world and that normal people are hearing people. We take it for granted that if a person is spoken to he will make an appropriate reply, that he will take evasive action if we sound our car horn and that he will respond to the telephone or door bell. When a hearing-impaired person deviates from such norms, his handicap will be seen as something discreditable. He will become aware of this 'stigma' when an employer turns him down or people with normal hearing tend to adopt a superior role or to display pity or impatience. The stigma is accentuated by the general tendency to label everyone with a hearing loss as 'deaf', irrespective of its extent or time of onset. There is also an unfortunate belief that in some ways deafness is related to daftness; too often the deaf and hard of hearing are stereotyped as slow-thinking and deficient in intelligence. Deafness, unlike blindness, is not a disability that makes an instinctive appeal to human sympathy. it is significant that while the deaf are usually found in comedies the blind appear in tragedies!

E. Goffman in *Stigma—Notes on the Management of Spoiled Identity* has stated that the rewards of being considered normal are so great that all handicapped people in a position to do so will, on occasion, attempt to bluff themselves off as 'normal'. Since, unlike the blind or crippled, hearing-impaired people display no external symptoms, there is a strong temptation to resort to subterfuges. Frances Warfield has given some amusing examples (in *There's No Need to Shout*) of the covers she adopted at football games to disguise the fact that she was hard of hearing: 'be chilly and muffle ears comically in scarf and lap robe; have foot go to sleep and create noise and laughter by stamping; divert escort's attention to getting and consuming of hot dogs, etc; do tricks with matches or handkerchiefs and encourage escort to do the same, tear up programmes; make and sail paper darts.' And at dances, she suggests: continue to sing tune last played; ask to be shown new dance step; play cagey and pretend you won't answer questions—you know the answer but you're not telling; read your partner's palm; powder your nose; lose something; remember you have to go to the telephone; ask for some punch.

This desire to pass as normal also explains the reluctance of many hard-of-hearing people to wear a hearing aid; they regard it as a stigma symbol advertising their disability. The wish for concealment is, of course, recognized by the hearing-aid manufacturers, both at the design stage when some efficiency in performance may be sacrificed in the interest of making the aid as small as possible, and in advertising when stress is laid on the aid's inconspicuousness. In short, bluffing is a desperate attempt by an individual threatened with being, or being thought, abnormal to retain the status and acceptability of a 'normal' person. When bluffing is no longer possible, or the strain of keeping up the pretence of normalcy becomes too great, the hearing-impaired person will tend to resort to withdrawal from society.

COPING WITH THE EMOTIONAL EFFECTS

It is easier to write about the effects of hearing impairment on personality and behaviour, and their causes, than to suggest just how they may be avoided or overcome. Your adjustment, or your friend's or relative's adjustment, to loss of hearing depends not only on the cause, severity and expected progress of the disability, but also on such variables as age, intelligence, personality, education and support received from family, friends and employers. In making suggestions as to how to cope, it is impossible to avoid generalizations. There is also the danger that a reader, facing the harsh reality of impaired hearing, may dismiss such generalizations as platitudinous preaching. The answer to that charge is that what follows is based not on idle theorizing but on some twenty years' personal experience of hearing impairment. This experience led to the conclusion that if one is to modify the emotional and behavioural effects of hearing loss it is necessary to cultivate at least five virtues: knowledge, honesty, empathy, activity and courage.

Knowledge. The fact that one's ears are dull is no reason why one's mind should not be active. A hearing-impaired person should try to discover, through reading and conversation with others, as much as possible about his handicap and the procedures, devices and agencies that may exist for its relief. At the simplest level such information will make him aware of such gadgets as the flashing door bells and other devices mentioned in Chapter 7. Knowledge about the possible results of hearing loss on behaviour can also prevent some embarrassing situations. For example people with a conductive loss tend to speak softly; those with a sensorineural loss are prone to shout. Knowing this simple fact will enable a person to modulate his voice appropriately. Being aware that 'substitute aggression' is a negative response to frustration may help an individual to curb any tendency to relieve his tension by venting his frustrations on others. Knowledge enables the handicapped to evaluate information and an informed person is much less likely to be taken in by charlatans offering wonder-cures. The very fact that you are reading this page indicates a desire to know something about hearing impairment. This attitude of curiosity and desire for understanding should be maintained.

Honesty. Honesty in this context means a firm resolve to avoid bluffing. No hearing-impaired person can bluff for very long, and even the attempt may make him appear ridiculous and involve unnecessary strain. Most people will be too polite to tell him that they are aware of his impairment and will allow him to believe that the bluff is succeeding when, in fact, he is fooling no one. It is much better to admit to a disability at the outset. If you cannot hear what is being said, the sensible thing is to explain simply and courteously that you don't hear well. The vast majority of people will then do all they can to help, and the minority who are impatient or ignorant can usually be ignored.

Most hearing-impaired people are more self-conscious than they need be. This point can be illustrated by a personal experience. After the first of two successful stapedectomy operations I returned to work and proudly asked a number of colleagues 'do you notice anything different?', expecting them to say at once 'You're not wearing your hearing aid.' To my surprise they scrutinized me closely and then admitted that they could not detect anything unusual. They had long since ceased even to notice the aid which I had thought to be so conspicuous.

Empathy. Empathy is the ability to identify with others. Empathy helps in making allowance for any conduct and attitudes from others that arise from ignorance and misunderstanding. Thus, at the beginning of this chapter it was stated that few people with normal ears are aware of the emotional and behavioural consequences of impaired hearing. It is also true that some people shy away from all types of handicap because they are embarrassed and uncertain what to do. In such cases, empathy enables the handicapped person to take the initiative and put the non-handicapped at ease by informing them how they can best assist. A person with a severe hearing loss might explain 'there is no need to shout, but if you will face the light and speak slowly I shall probably understand what you are saying.' Empathy leads to the realization that even the most patient husband or wife will also experience strain from having to act as a second pair of ears for a partner with defective hearing. It is all too easy for a hard-of-hearing person to become so full of self-pity that he is oblivious to the needs, difficulties and rights of others. A television set turned on at full volume can turn a home into a hell for everyone else there. A hearing-impaired person has to try to extend the same understanding to others that he expects to receive.

Activity. The best method of counteracting depression and social isolation is to cultivate some physical or mental activity—dealt with more fully in Chapter 9. It may be mentioned here that activity can divert the mind away from the disability and thereby prevent the introspection that so often results in depression.

Courage. Alfred Adler, the great Viennese psychologist, maintained that physical defects, whether congenital or acquired, invariably result in feelings of inferiority. These feelings, which often arise from the reduced ability of the disabled person to compete and interact with the non-handicapped, may also be reinforced by social attitudes. Unless a handicapped person is alert to the possibility he tends to become what he is expected to be. A person who, because of his impaired hearing, is regarded by his family and associates as dull and slow may come to regard these valuations as true. He will gradually develop an inferiority complex and fatalistically resign himself to a crippling situation which he will make no attempt to correct or improve. He may even attempt to exploit his ascribed inferiority to claim attention or gain sympathy. Aggression, self-assertion and rebellion may also be negative responses to inferiority.

A more constructive approach to overcoming inferiority is to find a compensation. Compensation involves finding out what can be done well and doing it. Thus a hearing-impaired person can compensate for any feeling of inferiority by channelling his energies into some activity that provides scope for demonstrating competence. For Adler (*Problems of Neurosis*) the decisive factor in determining whether an individual would succumb to or overcome inferiority was courage:

> By courage and training disabilities may be so compensated that they even become great abilities. When correctly encountered a disability becomes a stimulus that impels towards a higher achievement. . . . Those who have attained remarkable success in life have often been handicapped in the beginning with

disabilities and with great feelings of inferiority. On the other hand we find that a person who believes himself to be the victim of inherited deficiencies and disabilities lessens his efforts with a feeling of hopelessness and his development is thus permanently retarded.

Of the three possible attitudes to hearing impairment—rebellion, resignation and redemption—it is only the latter that, like Wordsworth's Happy Warrior 'turns necessity to glorious gain', yields positive results. Through years of depression and anxiety two quotations were a constant source of inspiration. The first states that 'character is a measure of the things that one has overcome'. The second is a prayer by Reinhold Niebuhr:

'God give me the serenity to accept the things I cannot change, the courage to change the things I can, and the wisdom to know the difference.'

7 Hearing Aids and Other Devices

The oldest, cheapest and most readily accessible aid to hearing is the cupped hand behind the ear. By channelling more sound-energy into the ear via the cupped hand the sound level at the ear can be raised by about six decibels. Many other ingenious aids have been devised to assist those with impaired hearing. M. A. Goldstein, in an historical survey (*Problems of the Deaf*) has classified hearing devices into the following six groups: hearing tubes; ear trumpets; concealed or camouflaged sound receptors, eg acoustic chairs, fans, hats, hair combs, walking sticks etc; devices to increase the size and capacity of parts of the sound-conducting mechanism, eg artificial external ears (auricles) and artificial ear-drums; non-electric bone-conduction devices, eg strips of wood, metal or vulcanite to conduct sound through the skull; electronic aids.

Some of the appliances that have been marketed have been valueless, and even callous, attempts to exploit the desperate desire of severely disabled people to hear as inconspicuously as possible. Other devices, especially hearing tubes and ear trumpets, rendered real assistance and are still useful particularly for those elderly people who find it difficult to adapt themselves to electronic aids. It is also possible to make a hearing tube at very little cost by purchasing about three feet of 10mm bore rubber tube from a chemist and pushing a small plastic or metal funnel into one end for speaking into. Although an earpiece is not strictly necessary it is possible to buy a suitable one from some hearing-aid dealers or even from radio shops.

It is, however, an electronic hearing aid that most people think about when considering how they can compensate for a loss of hearing. Although Alexander Graham Bell was seeking to make an electric hearing aid for his wife when, in 1876, he invented the magnetic telephone, it was not until 1898 that such an instrument was marketed in America by the Dictograph Company.

The first electric hearing aids were very cumbersome and it was only shortly before World War II that 'monopack' instruments appeared. The reduction in the size of hearing aids has been made possible by the development of miniature radio valves and by the transistor. Solid-state printed circuitry has been another important factor.

Below, something of the types and construction of instruments, and how an aid may be acquired, used and maintained, is explained. Reference will also be made to some other devices that may help a hearing-impaired person.

TYPES OF HEARING AIDS

Electronic hearing aids for personal use are available in an extensive variety of makes and models and over a wide price range. They may also be described in many ways. Some idea of what is available is provided by the 'List of Current Hearing Aids' published by and obtainable from the Royal National Institute for the Deaf. The list current at the time of writing gives details of 305 different commercial aids produced by 26 manufacturers and ranging in price (exclusive of the ear mould) from £46 to £362. In addition, particulars are given of 5 models available under the National Health Service.

Body-worn Aids

As the name implies, these are attached to the clothing. Because body-worn aids are larger than ear-level instruments it is possible for designers to provide higher levels of amplification and a wider frequency range, together with more sophisticated controls. Body-worn aids are, therefore, particularly suitable for people with severe hearing loss who require greater maximum output and acoustic gain than can normally be provided by an ear-level aid.

Ear-level Aids

While body aids have advantages for people with severe loss, ear-level aids are the choice for a person with a mild to moderate impairment. They include aids worn behind the ear (for either air conduction or bone conduction), those worn in the ear, and also spectacle aids—again either for air conduction or bone conduction. They offer the following advantages: they are considerably smaller than body aids; distortion arising from the rubbing of clothes against the microphone is eliminated; the ear-level aid is less conspicuous and, with women, can be completely concealed by an appropriate hair-style; the microphone is placed at ear level.

Behind-the-ear Aids. These are very inconspicuous and may have the microphone facing forwards or rearwards. For most hearing situations the forward-facing microphone is the most effective.

Spectacle Aids. These have the microphone, amplifier and receiver located in either one or both of the arms of the frame. Binaural hearing can be provided if the aid is in both arms. This arrangement is preferable to two body-worn aids as it allows natural head movements. The frames are also ideal for use in connection with 'bi-unilateral' hearing aids. These, known by the acronyms CROS and BICROS, are designed to assist people with a hearing loss in one ear or those who have little or no residual hearing in one ear and impaired hearing in the other. The primary goal is to improve the hearing of speech originating on the side of the weaker ear. The effect is to give the user a form of binaural hearing even where one ear is non-functional. He can then more easily tell from which direction a sound is coming.

CROS stands for contralateral routing of signals. In a unilateral loss, a CROS aid sends sounds from a microphone placed behind the bad ear to a receiver in the good ear. Spectacle frames provide an ideal carrying medium for the wire connecting the microphone to the receiver. BICROS, or bilateral contra-lateral routing of signals, is for people who have a bilateral loss with usable residual hearing in only one ear. In this system two microphones are used. The sounds picked up by the microphones are fed into a mixer unit that combines them before amplifying and transmitting them into the usable ear. One serious disadvantage of BICROS is that a great deal of sound is fed into the better ear, and where the loss in that ear is not great the user may complain that the reception is too loud.

Perhaps the most serious disadvantage of spectacle aids is their high cost. Single aids mounted in spectacle frames cost from about £120 upwards (at the time of writing), exclusive of lenses and ear-mould. A binaural aid would be approximately double the price. Some manufacturers do, however, provide spectacle arms that enable many behind-the-ear aids to be used as spectacle aids. These attachments are comparatively cheap. Details of suppliers are given in the RNID 'List of Current Hearing Aids'.

All-in-the-ear Aids. Often described as hearing correctors or clarifiers, these are very small since the entire aid pushes directly into the ear passage. A typical aid of this type measures 0.82×0.42×0.5in (2.1×1.1×1.3cm). The reduction in size, however, means some corresponding reduction in performance. Thus, while body-worn and behind-the-ear aids are capable of providing gains of up to 90 and 70 db respectively, the highest gain to the writer's knowledge, with an all-in-the-ear instrument is 45 db. These are therefore appropriate for borderline cases who might require an aid in some situations, eg meetings. All-in-the-ear aids are not invisible and, in fact, may be more conspicuous than a behind-the-ear aid. Sometimes the advertising matter put out by dealers and manufacturers does not stress the limitations of these aids sufficiently.

Binaural Aids

Where hearing aids are concerned, true binaural hearing means the use of two instruments. It does not mean just two earpieces connected by a Y-shaped cord to one aid. In theory two aids which only provide binaural *listening* should be better than one, for people with impaired hearing on both sides, since they should give some of the advantages of binaural hearing—especially improved sound location and discrimination in noisy conditions. But research reports on the advantages of binaural over monaural aids are inconclusive in their findings. A number of aid users have told me that from time to time they have worn an aid in each ear with some benefit, particularly if listening to music when the stereophonic effect has been enjoyed. The commonsense approach when considering the question of binaural versus monaural aids is to select whichever you find most beneficial, and whichever your otologist and your pocket prefer, in that order. Usually it is best to become accustomed to one aid before experimenting with two. Certainly a binaural aid should be given an extended trial before purchase.

THE COMPONENTS OF A HEARING AID

Many hearing-impaired people are unable to make the best use of information provided by manufacturers about hearing aids, or to hold informed discussions with salesmen, because they do not know the basic principles of hearing-aid construction.

Essentially a hearing aid is an amplifying device. Like any

other amplifying device it has four main components: a microphone, an amplifier, an earphone and the power supply. The ear mould, while not strictly part of the aid, is also an important element in its efficiency.

The Microphone. The purpose of the microphone is to change the energy carried by the sound waves into electrical energy. This is done by means of a diaphragm which is made to vibrate by the sound waves, very much like the ear-drum in the human ear.

The Amplifier. With its complicated assortment of transistors, capacitators, resistors and wires, the amplifier has the function of increasing the electrical voltage received by the microphone.

The Earphone. The earphone reverses the function of the microphone. Where the microphone changes sound waves into electrical energy the earphone transduces the electrical energy back again. Most earphones are air-conductive and feed into the ear passage by means of an ear mould. Where there is ear discharge or a very significant bone-air gap, a bone-conduction receiver may be fitted. A bone-conduction earphone is essentially a vibrator, which is placed against the mastoid so that sound can be transmitted into the inner ear. The disadvantage of bone-conduction earphones, which are limited to body and spectacle aids, is that they require more power with a subsequent increase in battery consumption, they transmit a narrower range of frequencies and, in body-aids, a headband must be worn to ensure an adequate amount of pressure on the mastoid. Unless properly fitted this may cause considerable discomfort.

The Power Supply. The battery is the heart of the hearing aid since it provides the power. Hearing-aid batteries fall into three broad categories.

Carbon-zinc batteries, similar to those used in pocket torches, have the advantage of a low initial cost but are not rechargeable. Their output declines gradually and some warning is therefore given to the user before the battery is completely spent.

In very small aids and correctors, *mercury or 'mallory' type batteries* are used. Although the initial cost is higher than for their carbon-zinc counterparts, mercury batteries work out cheaper in terms of hours per unit of cost. Mercury batteries do not fade gradually but maintain a uniform voltage until almost all the energy has been consumed; some users find the absence of warning before the cut out a disadvantage. Mercury cells can be recharged if not completely run down, but if heated to a high temperature too quickly or exposed to excessive recharging voltages they may burst dangerously. They should, therefore, never be 'cooked' in an oven and, even with a charge current, less than 1mA must be used.

The third type of battery is the genuinely *rechargeable cell*, made of combinations of metal such as nickel and cadmium or silver and zinc. Such cells do not generate electricity but absorb current from a battery charger in much the same way as a car battery accumulates current from the dynamo. These cells can be recharged up to 100 times and will last for about twelve months. Even though initially it is necessary to buy four batteries—one for the aid, one to keep in reserve, and two to be kept on charge—they are the most economical way of running a hearing aid over a period of a year. It should be remembered, however, that rechargeable batteries have to be changed more frequently than carbon-zinc or mercury types and some users do not think that the saving in cost compensates for the additional trouble involved.

Nickel-cadmium cells are obtainable from Birnatone Ltd, Watford, who also manufacture both a mains charger and a pocket battery charger smaller than a packet of ten cigarettes. Silver-zinc cells and the special charger for them can be bought from Medicharge Ltd, Watford. Information regarding all three varieties of battery is contained in an excellent pamphlet *Aids to Hearing* obtainable from the RNID. If you use carbon-zinc or mercury types it is a good idea to check the state of your batteries daily and the RNID pamphlet also gives details of a cheap but effective battery tester developed by the Institute.

The Ear Mould. The importance of the ear mould cannot be overstressed, since its design and fit can significantly influence the performance of the aid. The frequency response of the aid will be affected by the size and shape of the mould channel through which sound is fed into the outer ear. Unless an airtight fit is secured there will be an uncomfortable and embarrassing whistling from the aid due to feed-back.

Ear moulds are made individually from an impression of your ear passage and auricle. Technicians do not always get the mould right first time. You should not be afraid to refuse to accept a mould which is uncomfortable or is responsible for acoustic feed-back. A preparation known as Otoform Comfort Cream which makes moulds more comfortable and improves the seal is available from some hearing-aid dealers.

Hearing-aid Controls

Hearing-aid salesmen sometimes become almost lyrical about the wonderful controls of their instruments. To avoid being blinded with science you should be able to recognise the names of these controls and know what they are designed to do.

The Volume Control (VC). This control is more accurately called the 'Gain Control' since it controls amplification (gain) rather than loudness. 'Gain' may be defined as the output of the aid at the receiver minus the input at the microphone. If at 1,000 Hz the output of the aid is 100 db and the input 60 db then, at the given frequency, the gain is 40 db. The user can move the volume control to any of up to ten positions, thus regulating the amplifier's output according to the extent of his impairment or the amount of background noise.

Automatic Volume Control (AVC). Excessively loud sounds can cause distortion and even pain to the wearer of an aid. The function of the AVC is to limit the maximum output of the amplifier so that, irrespective of the input level, the output can never exceed a predetermined volume which is below the user's pain threshold.

Peak Clipping (PC). Like AVC this is a method of limiting the maximum output of the amplifier. By this method peak intensities are cut off whenever they exceed a pre-set output limit. It is known that the loss in the intelligibility of speech is insignificant when the peak intensities of sound are not transmitted by an aid. Nearly all aids have some form of peak clipping.

Dynamic Range Compression (DRC). Like AVC and Peak Clipping, DRC is intended to control sound pressures to a level below that at which discomfort and distortion is experienced. Unlike AVC and PC which are limited to a fixed *output* sound pressure, DRC is linked to a fixed *input* sound pressure level. DRC which is incorporated in the more expensive aids is particularly useful in cases of sensorineural impairment when recruitment is pronounced.

Tone Control (TC). This is a control designed to modify either the high or low frequencies. If the switch is set in the 'high' position less amplification will be given to the low and mid-frequencies. In the 'low' position the high frequencies will be reduced.

Telephone Coil. The correct term is 'inductive pick-up coil'. When the switch is in the T (telephone) position the microphone is automatically disconnected and only the pick-up coil is operative. The user of the aid can therefore listen exclusively to the telephone, extraneous sounds being eliminated. Other settings are M, when the microphone only is connected, and MT, in which both microphone and pick-up coil are operational.

THE NATIONAL HEALTH AID AND HOW TO GET ONE

Due to the advocacy of the then President of the RNID, the Duke of Montrose, the Medresco hearing aid was included among the list of appliances which may be issued on free loan under the provisions of the National Health Service Act of 1946.

At the time of writing the full range of Medresco aids is as follows:

TYPE NUMBER	TONE CONTROL	PICK-UP COIL	PRE-SET OUTPUT CONTROL	RECEIVERS	DEGREE OF HEARING LOSS	CHILD OR ADULT
OL56	no	no	yes	OL575 OL675	average more severe	adult
OL57	no	yes	yes	as above	as above	child
OL58*	no	yes	no	bone conductor	conductive loss	adult or child
OL63*	yes	no	no	OL575 OL675 OL375	average more severe very severe	adult or child
OL67 (Behind the Ear)	yes (pre-set)	yes	no	OL695 OL685	moderate loss lower loss	child
BE11	yes	yes	no	—	moderate	adult or child
BE12	no	yes	no	—	moderate	adult or child

* These aids will be replaced by an improved instrument in 1978

At present all the aids other than the OL67, BE11 and BE12 are body-worn and look alike. The aid most usually issued to adults is the OL56 but behind-the-ear aids will no doubt become the standard issue as they become more available.

To obtain a Medresco the first step is to tell your doctor that you wish to obtain an NHS aid. You will then be referred to an otologist, who will examine your ears to see whether an aid is appropriate. If you could be helped by surgical treatment, you will be given the choice of an aid or an operation, and if you decide on the latter you may be provided with an aid as an interim measure. On the basis of his examination and audiometric tests, the otologist will recommend the Medresco aid most suitable for your use. With the aid you will receive an initial supply of batteries, a booklet of instructions and a record book in which details of subsequent issues of batteries or repairs will be entered. Should the aid require attention you simply return it to the centre at which it was issued, and a minor repair will be done while you wait. If it cannot be done at once you will be provided with a replacement. This service is one of the major advantages of owning a NHS aid.

Although some commercial suppliers do lend aids to specially favoured customers, they obviously cannot keep a sufficient range in stock to meet the demands of all clients who need to be tided over a repair period. It is also advisable to find out the reference numbers of commercially available batteries equivalent to the CPI and other NHS aid batteries so that you can buy them from an electrical dealer should you need them at weekends or to avoid travelling to the hearing-aid clinic.

Finally, it must be stressed that all NHS aids are *lent*, not given, and that if for any reason you no longer require your instrument it should be returned without delay.

COMMERCIAL AIDS

A report on hearing aids published by *Which?* in 1973 included a survey of about 1,000 people who possessed both a Medresco and a commercial aid. Opinion on which aid provided better hearing was divided equally. When asked to express a preference, however, 60 per cent chose their commercial aid, against 30 per cent for the Medresco. Some bias in these returns probably arose from the fact that at the time of the survey only body-aids were available under the NHS and behind-the-ear commercial models were often preferred because they were less conspicuous, avoided clothes rub, were more comfortable to wear and easier to use. As behind-the-ear aids become generally obtainable under the Health Service it is possible that the much greater popularity of commercial instruments will be reduced.

There are two main advantages in owning both a Medresco

and a commercial aid. Firstly you are insured against the embarrassment of being without an instrument should one require repair. Secondly, Medresco aids are designed to meet the requirements of the majority of users and the range of choice is therefore small in contrast to the wide variety of commercial aids. An informative price list sent to the writer by a large London hearing-aid dealer gives details of 32 behind-the-ear, 12 body, 12 spectacle and 1 in-the-ear instruments. Particulars are provided of the suitability of each aid for losses of from 30 to 90 db and instruments suitable for conditions such as recruitment are indicated. It should be possible for such a dealer to fit an aid more closely suited to your particular requirements, another factor to influence users towards commercial aids. Before rushing out to buy one, however, you should pause to consider the likely cost involved.

The truth that the ability to hear without strain cannot be measured in monetary terms should not blind us to the high capital and running costs incurred in the purchase and use of a hearing aid. At the time of writing, the price range varies from £49 to £320, to which about £6 must be added for the ear mould. The running costs are often assumed to comprise only expenditure on batteries and repairs, but a truer picture would include such items as depreciation, insurance and loss of interest on a capital investment of, say, £130.

Battery life is a very significant factor, and it is important to remember that the 'life' can vary significantly according to the type of aid. Thus in a price list battery lives vary from 28 to 1,000 hours. The life of an MP675H battery is specified as being from 140 to 500 hours. This variation in life is accounted for by the varying amounts of power required for different degrees of hearing loss. When the aid is on 'low' a life of 500 hours will be obtained; where maximum power is needed the life is reduced to 140 hours. Let us assume that for medium output the life will be 300 hours and that the aid will be in use for 15 hours daily. You will therefore require a new battery every 20 days or 18 batteries per year. At the time of writing the MP675H battery costs 96p so that your annual outlay would be £17.28.

Repairs are difficult to forecast. All reputable manufacturers guarantee their instruments for at least the first 12 months and sometimes longer. Minor repairs such as cords and the replacement of the plastic ear tubes are relatively cheap. Other repairs can be very expensive especially where the dealer has to return the aid to the manufacturer. One dealer made an analysis of the cost of 50 major repairs undertaken in June 1976. The average cost of each repair was £13.39 and a more detailed breakdown was as follows: Under £10, 24 per cent; £10–£16, 50 per cent; £16–£20, 12 per cent; £20–£26, 14 per cent. We can assume that £20 (at current rates) will be spent on repairs of all types during the life of an aid.

The life of the aid will, of course, depend on its usage. Aids may be considered to have a life of approximately 5–7 years. At 15 hours' use per day, five years is the safer estimate and at the end of that time the question of replacement will arise. Most dealers will allow a nominal trade-in for an old aid to someone buying a new one. The annual depreciation charge will be determined by the total cost of the aid, say £130, less the trade-in, say £15, divided by the life (say 5 years), which works out at £23.

A hearing aid is a valuable instrument and it is advisable to insure it against loss or theft. Premiums are not high and an annual figure of £3.06 was quoted by one insurance broker.

Finally, if you did not require an aid or relied exclusively on the Medresco you could invest your purchase price of £130 in a building society and, at the standard rate, obtain a tax-free return of $6\frac{1}{2}$ per cent or £8.45 per annum! The realistic annual cost of using the specified commercial aid would work out at £56.79 or £1.09 per week, being the cost of the batteries plus the repairs, depreciation, insurance and loss of interest from money spent on the aid which could otherwise have been invested. This cost, can, of course, be reduced by using your commercial aid at work and your Medresco at home. The cost will also tend to be higher in the later years of the aid's life.

As an alternative to outright purchase some hearing-aid dealers operate rental schemes. One drawback of these is that a dealer can only keep a limited range of aids available for rental. Since this range will tend to cater for 'run-of-the-mill' cases of hearing impairment, the most suitable aid for you may well not be included in the selection available. Do not, therefore, enter into a rental agreement until you have tried out some other aids. Another point to bear in mind is that some rental agreements require the aid to be retained for several years. Since you may be entering into a fairly long-term contract you should scrutinize the agreement, especially the small print, very carefully before committing yourself in writing. In particular you should seek written clarification on such matters as these:

    For what period is the rental payable?

    What are the provisions for cancellation of the rental agreement before the agreed termination date?

    What is covered by the rental, eg the aid only or the aid plus batteries and repairs?

    Are there any limitations on what is provided under the agreement?

    What rights does the hirer retain to increase the rental or assign the contract?

    Whose liability is it should the aid be stolen or damaged?

    Are there any provisions for exchanging the aid for a newer or more suitable model during the period of the rental agreement?

Buying a Commercial Aid

It is not difficult to find a 'dispenser of hearing aids'. The yellow pages of a telephone directory will usually provide a selection of dealers willing to supply you. Suppliers of aids also make extensive use of press advertising to bring their wares to the notice of prospective users. Before trying to find a dealer, however, you would be wise to do two things. Firstly, if you have not already done so, ask your doctor to refer you to an otologist. This advice is worth reiterating, since it may be that appropriate treatment would remove the need for an aid. Secondly, if you *do* need an aid, start by writing to the RNID and asking for their list of hearing aids. This publication will provide you with particulars of the names, descriptions and prices of the majority of hearing aids on the market.

It is also worth bearing in mind the finding reported in the *Which?* survey of 1973 that 'people whose choice of a dealer was based on a recommendation by a friend, relation or doctor were, on average, more satisfied than people who had chosen from an advertisement'. If you do not wish a representative to call at your home when you reply to an advertisement, say so when making the enquiry, thereby saving the salesman's time and your own. Apart from this general advice some of the following hints may also be useful.

    Try to locate a dealer within reasonable distance of your home to save unnecessary expense and inconvenience should your aid require after-sales service.

    Don't buy from a travelling exhibition unless the supplier can provide acceptable after-sales facilities within your area.

    Tell the dispenser the type of aid you would prefer, eg behind-the-ear, spectacle, etc and how much you wish to pay. Let him know when the aid will usually be worn, eg in the home, in a noisy factory, etc.

A good dispenser will test your ability to discriminate speech sounds as well as pure tones. The *Which?* survey reported that less than half of their respondents had been tested by speech audiometry.

Do not expect a hearing-aid dispenser to prescribe with the same precision as an optician. He will generally categorize your loss as 'mild', 'moderate' or 'severe' and select aids from his stock which he believes to be appropriate.

Make allowances for some distortion and oscillation when you try an aid with a *standard* ear mould. An *individual* ear mould will almost certainly improve reception.

Before purchasing ask the dispenser whether you may try the aid for a few days at home, either free or on the basis of a returnable deposit. If a trial on such terms is refused you are well advised not to buy. While the aid is in your possession treat it carefully, test it fairly and, if you decide not to purchase, return it promptly either in person or by registered post.

Only *you* can decide which aid is the most satisfactory from the standpoints of comfort, speech intelligibility and tone quality. Do not be master-minded into buying any other aid.

Do not pay more than you need for an aid. Ask about discount, particularly if you are paying cash. If you have previously used a hearing aid ascertain whether the dispenser will give a 'trade-in' for your old instrument. The allowance will be small, but a useful contribution to the cost of your new aid.

When purchasing an aid it is reasonable to expect one year's guarantee covering repairs.

CONSUMER PROTECTION AND THE HEARING-AID USER

In 1964 a writer in *The Silent World* wrote indignantly about 'the cruel and wicked methods' used by some hearing-aid manufacturers 'of forcing sales upon poor and hesitant purchasers' and 'high pressure salesmen with one foot in the door and their thumb across the penalty clause of a hire purchase agreement'. The gradual improvement in ethical standards of the sales and advertising methods relating to hearing aids has been achieved largely through the pioneer efforts of the RNID with some cooperation from within the industry itself.

The RNID still acts as a watchdog over the interests of the hearing-aid user, and through its Hearing Aid Advisory Service will provide free and unbiased advice to anyone who is contemplating the purchase of an aid. Aids and repairs to aids can also be tested and reported on, but not actually serviced, by the RNID Laboratory. The role of the RNID in protecting the user from unscrupulous sales methods or misleading advertising has now been largely taken over by the Hearing Aid Council and the Advertising Standards Authority.

The Hearing Aid Council was established by the Board of Trade in 1969 following the passing in the previous year of the Hearing Aid Council Act. The main statutory responsibilities of the Council are:

> 1. To provide for the registration with the Council of all dispensers selling hearing aids and all employers of such dispensers. It is now illegal for unregistered individuals, partnerships or companies to sell hearing aids. The Disciplinary Committee of the Council has power to remove the name of any registered person or body corporate from the register.
> 2. To lay down standards of competence for hearing-aid dispensers and those wishing to take up the occupation.
> 3. To lay down a Code of Trade Practice for adoption by registered dispensers and employees of dispensers. This Code is reproduced in Appendix 1.

When introducing the Hearing Aid Council Bill in 1968, Laurie Pavitt declared that his purpose was 'to protect the hard of hearing from the hard selling' and to 'put service, education and information in the place of gimmicky sales promotion'. There is little doubt that the Act has done much to achieve these objectives although some dealers are still not following the Code to the letter. The *Which?* survey of 1973 mentioned that although the Code requires a dispenser to ascertain whether a prospective client has seen a doctor before fitting an aid for the first time, 10 out of 45 new users reported that their dealer had not made this enquiry.

The Hearing Aid Council has no jurisdiction over hearing-aid advertisements. The only legal remedy against these lies in the Trade Descriptions Act. The Advertising Standards Authority has published the British Code of Advertising Practice, which lays down the following rules for advertisements relating to hearing aids and hearing-aid exhibitions:

> *8.17 Hearing Aids*
> 8.17.1 Where an advertisement states the price of a hearing aid, the advertiser should specify the upper and lower limits of his overall price range.

8.17.2 The names of hearing aids should not in themselves exaggerate the products effectiveness (eg such names as 'Magic Sound' and 'Miracle Ear' are not acceptable).

8.17.3 Advertisements for hearing aids on a rental basis are subject to the rules applying to hire of domestic appliances.

8.18 Hearing Aid Exhibitions

8.18.1 Advertisements for such exhibitions should only be accepted where the organiser has given an undertaking:
1. That he will ensure the presence of at least one registered dispenser at all times throughout the period the exhibition is open.
2. That he will offer for inspection a comprehensive range of models of hearing aids.
3. That he will make available for purposes of testing at least one pure tone *and* one speech audiometer.

8.18.2 The full name and address of the advertiser's head office should be prominently stated in any advertisement for a hearing aid show or exhibition, and no impression should be given that such events are other than commercially promoted.

If you have a complaint against a hearing-aid dispenser, or consider that you have been misled by an advertisement, the initial move is to take up the complaint personally or in writing with the dispenser or his employer. If you fail to obtain satisfaction report the circumstances with *copies* of supporting evidence to the Hearing Aid Council or Advertising Standards Authority whichever is appropriate. If the matter is still not resolved the only course is to seek legal remedies—not a thing to be done lightly and without sound professional advice.

THE USE AND MAINTENANCE OF AN AID

Whether you acquire a Medresco through the National Health Service, or invest some of your money in a commercial aid, you must not expect to obtain the maximum benefit immediately. Adjustment to a hearing aid is affected by many variables. The age and personality of the user, the cause and duration of the hearing loss, the suitability of the aid for a particular case and the environment in which the aid is used all influence the time necessary to adapt to it. Perseverance, commonsense and some understanding of the aid are essential. itself are essential.

Using the Aid

A booklet entitled *General Guidance to Hearing Aid Users* is issued with every Medresco aid. Some similar publication is usually given to the purchaser of a commercial aid. The following advice is intended to reinforce or supplement that given in such guides.

1. Recognize the limitations of your aid. Basically a hearing aid is an amplifying device. It will not wholly provide the clear discrimination, selectivity and location of sound that is obtained from normal hearing.

2. Recognize your own limitations. The fault may be in yourself rather than the aid. If your impairment is of long duration you may have become so conditioned to living in a quiet world that at first you resent rather than welcome the noise in your environment that becomes more audible with your aid. Older people may take longer to adjust than younger ones. Presbyacusis and other sensorineural conditions may be accompanied by recruitment, so that the margin between your SRT and the overloading of your cochlea is small. Fatigue, nerves and even minor illnesses such as a cold may adversely affect your reception.

3. Wear the earpiece of a monaural aid in the most *suitable* ear. Your otologist or hearing-aid dispenser will advise you on that; it is not necessarily the *better* ear as determined by a pure-tone test. If you have a loss greater than 60 db in both ears, the earpiece should be worn in the ear which is best for speech, as determined by the appropriate audiometric tests. Where the loss is dissimilar, say 40 db and 70 db in the right and left ears respectively, it is normally preferable to wear the earpiece in the poorer ear. The principle behind this advice is that with a loss of less than 60 db the better ear, if not blocked by the earpiece, can still perceive some speech naturally.

4. Learn lipreading if you have difficulty in discriminating speech sounds. As shown in the next chapter, lipreading may enhance the effectiveness of a hearing aid.

5. Wear the aid sensibly. Ideally a body-worn aid should have the microphone in the centre of the chest. Some men find it useful to wear the microphone inside the tie and to keep the cord in place by positioning it between the neck and the shirt collar. Women can wear the microphone under the dress in a pocket sewn to the centre of the bra. Both of these methods may result in some distortion arising from 'clothes rub' due to the movements of garments against the microphone. 'Clothes rub' can be eliminated by the use of a 'Medresco purse' obtainable very cheaply from the RNID. The purse consists of a suede

plastic pocket with a rustle-free lining into which a Medresco or aid of similar size fits snugly. A cotton cord enables the purse to be suspended from the neck of the wearer at a convenient height.

6. Use the controls intelligently. If you have difficulty in quiet surroundings you should turn up the volume. Conversely, if you are in noisy surroundings it is sensible to turn the volume down. Make use of the telephone coil when applicable.

Maintaining the Aid

The routine attention you can give to your aid is limited to the batteries, ear mould, cord (on body-worn aids) and the short plastic tube feeding into the channel of the ear mould on most behind-the-ear instruments. Batteries must be inserted correctly and always be of the type specified for the aid. Remove the batteries immediately they are spent or if you do not intend to use the aid for any length of time. The ear mould should be cleaned regularly by washing it in warm soapy water, removing any wax from the channel with a pipe-cleaner. The mould should, of course, first be detached from the earphone on a body-worn aid or the plastic tube on a behind-the-ear instrument. The plastic tube itself may eventually become stiff and even break, though its replacement on an aid is cheap and simple. Cords on body-worn aids also become brittle after a time and may then either distort reception or transmit no sound at all. Medresco aids are usually issued with a spare cord and if you use a commercial aid a spare cord should be kept in stock. In fact, a wise hearing-aid user carries with him an emergency pack of batteries, plastic tubing and spare cord (for body-worn aids only).

Looking after a hearing aid is largely a matter of common sense. The aid should be protected from moisture and heat. It should not, for example, be left on a hot radiator or exposed to hot sunshine. Obviously an aid will not be improved by being dropped, so you should ensure that it is securely fixed whenever you put it on.

Apart from the simple repairs described above you should never attempt to interfere with the interior of the aid. It is useful, however, to be able to identify possible faults and the following checklist may be helpful.

SOME COMMON HEARING-AID PROBLEMS

PROBLEM	ITEMS TO CHECK	POSSIBLE CAUSE	SUGGESTED ACTION
no sound	(a) ear mould	channel blocked with wax	clean ear mould
	(b) batteries	battery spent battery wrongly inserted battery contacts dirty	replace with new insert correctly clean – with a Medresco aid this must be done at a hearing-aid centre
	(c) plastic tube (on behind-the-ear aid)	condensation in the tube	remove the ear mould and blow through the tube but **NEVER INTO** the aid
	(d) cord (on body-worn aid)	cord broken or damaged	replace cord
	(e) earphone	faulty earphone or socket	ask hearing aid technician to confirm and if necessary replace
	(f) body of aid (on body-worn aid)	faulty socket	move cord in and out of socket. Return aid for repair
low output from aid	battery volume control	low-voltage battery wrong setting of volume control	replace battery correct setting
crackling	cord or cord plug socket (on body-worn aids)	damaged cord	replace cord
	battery	poor contact	clean exposed surface of battery with emery cloth or replace
	volume control	dirty volume control	return aid for cleaning of contacts or volume control, checking of sockets or other repairs
squealing or whistling	ear mould	poor fitting	ask technician to check fit

OTHER AIDS

Many hard-of-hearing people find that a hearing aid

83

enables them to cope satisfactorily with all the auditory requirements of daily life. There are others, however, who due to the type of severity of their hearing loss need additional help. A survey of people with hearing difficulties made in Blaby, Leicestershire (Skeikh and Verney, *Report on the Survey of Hearing Impaired Persons in Blaby*—Leicester County Council Social Services Department) called attention to the way in which many people could be helped by 'relatively simple technical aids':

> Many of the housewives described how they missed hearing door bells, thus annoying tradesmen and missing friends. On the occasion when a caller was expected, they described how they would stay in the front rooms of the house in order to see him; much anxiety would have been saved by a flashing-light door bell. One mother used to sit on the stairs in the hall when she was alone and her husband on night shift, so she could hear her children if they cried. A major source of tension in many households centred round television viewing. For some households television viewing is one of the main interests outside working hours, but at loud volume can disturb neighbours, children in bed, and irritate beyond measure normally hearing people in the family. The alternative means that the hard of hearing person is excluded. Once again a gadget could have saved many hours of tension.

The most comprehensive guide to some of the ingenious devices that have been produced to help the hearing impaired is the RNID publication *Special Aids to Hearing*, which the reader is urged to acquire since it gives details of the manufacturers concerned. These special aids may be considered under three main headings: radio and television; telephone; and visual aids.

Hearing Radio and Television

Many people with impaired hearing do not enjoy radio and television because of the inconvenience that a set turned up to maximum volume would cause to other members of their family or to neighbours. This difficulty can be overcome in several ways. Probably the simplest solution to the problem is by means of headphones connected to the radio or television receiver. It is important, however, to consider before purchase that the output of the headphones will be adequate for the needs of the user. The 'Varisona' radio receiver specially designed for people who are hard of hearing is described in *Special Aids to Hearing*.

Most hearing-aid dispensers stock special adaptors. These devices consist of a control box fitted at the back of the radio or television set in which a volume control is incorporated. Sound is fed to the listener by means of a cord to which an earpiece receiver is attached. This earpiece can be clipped to the user's ear mould. Some adaptors enable the television or radio to be switched on or off by remote control. For safety, adaptors must always be fitted by a qualified electrician.

A third method by which hearing-impaired people can enjoy radio or television without the embarrassment of annoying others is the inductive loop system, which enables a hearing aid fitted with an induction or telephone pick-up coil to pick up sound from transmitting stations. The 'loop', which can be fastened round the room or under the carpet, runs from and to the radio or television set. The inductive loop system has two outstanding advantages. It is cheap and easy to install, and it enables the hearing-aid user to listen to programmes while moving freely about the room. For television sets it is again important to stress that the installation should, for safety reasons, be left to a television engineer.

The Telephone

For personal and employment purposes the inability to use a telephone is a serious handicap. The Post Office is not unaware of this problem and has issued a descriptive leaflet DLE 550 entitled *Help for the Handicapped*. Its front page specifically points out that the Chronically Sick and Disabled Persons Act of 1970 empowers local authorities to provide, or assist in obtaining, a telephone or any necessary special equipment for the handicapped. In appropriate cases, eg for aged hard-of-hearing people living alone, it might be worth discussing the question of special equipment with the Social Services Department of your local authority. The same leaflet also carries the information that the Post Office wishes to ensure: 'That each handicapped person, and anyone in an organisation which sets out to assist them, is fully aware of each piece of our equipment, large or small, which can be of help.'

Anyone who is hearing-impaired and in the course of his daily work experiences difficulty with the telephone, might ask his employer to ascertain whether one of the Post Office instruments could be obtained to help him cope with the problem. While the five devices mentioned below are not free the installation and quarterly charges are very small.

The Amplifying Telephone Handset. This can be substituted for the normal telephone handset. The amplifying handset has a volume control in the side of the earpiece which enables the sound to be increased from normal to a level suitable to the requirements of the user.

The 'Watch' Receiver. This device, which is an additional earpiece, can be fitted to either a normal or amplified telephone, thus making it possible for the user to listen to telephone messages with both ears. Where a hearing aid incorporates a telephone coil the earpiece can also be held against the microphone of the aid, so that the user can listen through his hearing-aid earphone while speaking towards the transmitter of the handset in the usual way.

Extension Bells. These bells, which vary in loudness and tone, can be fitted wherever they would best be heard by people who have difficulty in hearing the normal call signal from the telephone.

The Trimphone. The little 'Trimphone' has a distinctive warbling tone which some hard-of-hearing people can detect more clearly than the sound of the normal telephone bell.

Lamp Signals. Flashing light signals can be used to alert a hearing-impaired person to incoming calls. One signal is a small flashing light in the back of the handset. Others available include a table lamp which flashes in conjunction with the ringing of the telephone. These devices are particularly useful in alerting a hard-of-hearing person to telephone calls received during television programmes.

Visual and Other Signals

The system of lamp signals used for the telephone can clearly be extended to assist the hard of hearing in other ways. An alternative to the visual signal is vibration. It would be impractical to discuss all these aids here, and the interested reader can obtain details from the RNID booklet mentioned earlier. The devices available include: light-flashing door-bells, warning doormats, visual baby alarms, flashing alarm clocks, vibrating fire alarms and vibrating alarm clocks.

All these contrivances, which are relatively inexpensive, should be more widely known. They can do much to reduce the strain and uncertainty of hearing impairment.

8 Lipreading

Almost everyone uses vision to supplement the information received through hearing and other senses. We all watch the face of a speaker when we have difficulty in hearing what is being said: even people with normal hearing may be unconscious lipreaders. But what is lipreading? What are its limitations and advantages? How can lipreading be learned and used in everyday situations?

THE BASIS OF LIPREADING

Lipreading is the reception of spoken messages through the medium of vision. An alternative term favoured in the USA and increasingly adopted in Britain is 'speechreading'. The advocates of speechreading hold that the term describes the process more accurately. Lipreading implies that only the lips of the speaker are observed. Speechreading recognizes that the reception of speech involves watching the jaws, tongue and total facial expression as well as the lips. Arguably both terms give the erroneous impression that speech can be read from the lips as easily as reading a book or newspaper. While speechreading may be the more technically correct expression, lipreading is the word that is most popularly understood and is therefore used here.

Basically lipreading is a skill involving three elements. Spoken language is composed of identifiable 'speech sounds' or small variations in air pressure that can be sensed by the ear. In English there are forty-odd speech sounds that are classified as shown on page 88.

Some speech sounds give rise to recognizable movements of the mouth, tongue and lips of the speaker. Thus, to give a few examples, vowel sounds such as 'ar' and 'aw' are made with the mouth wide open. For 'oo' and 'ee' the mouth opening is narrow.

ENGLISH SPEECH SOUNDS: CONSONANTS (26)

Vocals (14) (Those with voice)	Non-vocals (12) (Those with breath but no voice)
—	h
wh	w
f	u
p	b m
t	d n
th (as in though)	th (as in thin)
s	z
sh	zh
ch	j
k	g ng
x = rs	—
g = kwh	—
	v
	l

ENGLISH SPEECH SOUNDS: VOWELS (17)

Long Vowels	Short Vowels	Diphthongs
ar	oo (as in book)	ou
aw	u	ou
oo (as in soon)	o	oi
oe	a	ie
er	e	ae
ee	i	ew

(Table adapted from J. H. Burchett, *Lipreading*, 1965.)

To form 't', 'd' and 'n' we place the tip of the tongue to the upper gum. In the list above, 'p', 'b' and 'm' are grouped together because they are made by compressing the lips, 'f' and 'v' involve placing the lower lip against the top teeth while 'sh' is formed by pushing out the lips.

Where speech sounds cannot be distinguished on the lips, the lipreader has to deduce the appropriate sound or words from the general context of the message. Speech sounds or words may be unrecognizable for several reasons. While in one second about thirteen articulatory movements are made by the average speaker, the eye of the receiver is capable of consciously recording eight or nine such movements. Approximately 25 per cent of all the sounds produced are therefore missed by the eye. In fact, the number of speech movements missed is greater since not all sounds are visible in the first place. Jeffers and Barley consider that only four out of fourteen identifiable lipreading movements can be consistently recognized under normal viewing conditions 'the visibility of the remaining movements varying with the speaker, the rate of speech and the transitional characteristics of the speech patter'. In addition, many sounds and words are 'homopheneous'. This means that sounds or words look alike on the lips of the speaker. No lipreader can distinguish between 'p', 'b' and 'm' since, as stated above, they all involve the same lip movements. The only way in which the difficulty can be overcome is to link the word with its context. In ordinary circumstances we have to decide whether to understand 'wear' or 'where' or 'tire' or 'tyre' from the context. Similarly, a lipreader has to choose between 'Ben', 'men' and 'pen' to complete the sentence 'he had ten thousand . . .' Clearly the choice of 'men' is made as being the most appropriate alternative. Lipreading is thus not merely a matter of watching speech movements but of considerable mental effort in making sense from an incompletely perceived message.

LIMITATIONS AND ADVANTAGES OF LIPREADING

Lipreading has other limitations apart from relying on a considerable element of educated guesswork. Its usefulness is confined to speech. It offers no help with music, bird songs or warning signals. It is only of limited value in group conversation and useless if the speaker is behind or out of the range of vision of the lipreader. Furthermore lipreading is tiring because it demands intense concentration. Why then attempt to learn a skill which has so many drawbacks even for the very proficient? The answer is that many people with a severe hearing impairment have found lipreading to be a worthwhile accomplishment which has amply repaid the time and effort devoted to learning it.

How lipreading may increase the usefulness of a hearing aid was demonstrated by a series of experiments at Manchester University as long ago as 1943. These experiments involved ninety unselected persons aged from 17 to 72 who had an acquired hearing impairment. Eighty-seven of the participants had attended classes in lipreading. The purpose of the experiment was to ascertain the benefits that the group members had obtained from lipreading and hearing aids. The following results were reported:

CONDITIONS OF TEST	AVERAGE SCORE PER CENT
Ordinary listening without hearing aid or lipreading	21
Ordinary listening with lipreading	64
Listening with an electronic aid without lipreading	64
Listening with an electronic aid together with lipreading	90

(Ewing, Sir Alexander and Lady E. C. *Hearing Aids, Lipreading and Clear Speech*)

The advantages of combining the use of an aid with lipreading have been confirmed by later experiments.

Lipreading can be an important psychological help for a person faced by a sudden and severe irreversible hearing impairment. Learning lipreading is one of the few positive steps that people in these circumstances can take towards rehabilitation, and the effort required may assist in reducing depression. Lipreading can also reduce the sense of social isolation. When asked to name the greatest benefit she had received from a series of lessons in lipreading a lady replied 'I am no longer afraid to go shopping.'

You should give serious consideration to learning lipreading: where you have a sensorineural or mixed sensorineural/conductive loss, or a progressive conductive loss that cannot be treated by surgery; where the degree of loss is 70 db or greater over the speech frequencies; where the usefulness of a hearing aid is reduced by difficulties in discrimination.

LEARNING TO LIPREAD

The best way of learning lipreading is to join a class, where you have the guidance of a teacher and the stimulus of fellow students. Apart from large towns, however, a lipreading class may not be easy to find. Your hearing-aid centre may be able to help, and both the RNID and the BAHOH will, on request, provide a list of lipreading classes of which they have been notified. Local education authorities can sometimes arrange for instruction in lipreading at an evening institute or college of further education, especially if you can find six to eight people all interested in learning. In London, the hearing impaired are particularly fortunate, in that a Department of the Further Education of the Deaf has been established by the Inner London Education Authority as part of the work of the City Literary Institute. At Keeley House, Keeley Street, London WC2, it caters for four categories of students: those born with defective hearing; those who have acquired a hearing loss in adult life; students with speech defects unrelated to hearing; students whose work or family background brings them into contact with hearing impairment. Lipreading classes are provided in the morning, afternoon and evening, graded to cater for the whole range of lipreaders from beginners to advanced. Classes are purposely kept small.

If you join a lipreading class you will probably find that the teacher introduces both analytical and synthetical elements into the lesson. The purpose of the analytical element is to train the eyes of the lipreader to recognize speech sounds on the lips of the speaker. The aim of the synthetical element is to train the mind of the lipreader to grasp the total import of a message even though all the individual words are not recognized. An important part of the instruction will be designed to improve your ability to lipread at speed and to cope with colloquial language, different faces and varying situations. This instruction need not be dull and by using a variety of approaches and activities such as word games and group question-and-answer sessions, the good teacher can do much to make learning lively and even pleasurable.

No one would expect to become an expert pianist on the basis of one weekly session with a music teacher. Daily practice is needed if one is to become a proficient lipreader. You need a small mirror and a good friend. The mirror will enable you to see how speech sounds appear on your own lips. Your teacher will give you exercises to practice at home. Observing in a mirror the speech movements in a sentence such as 'Pa may we all go too' will give invaluable help in mastering the appropriate vowels. The friend can not only help with your exercises but also give additional practice with words, numbers and structured sentences. It is important to tell your friend to speak naturally and refrain from exaggerated 'mouthing'. You can also practice lipreading informally with your family at the breakfast table or by observing other people when standing in the bus queue. Television can provide excellent lipreading practice, though beginners may find that rapidly changing camera views make people too difficult to follow. When some proficiency has been attained, television can become much more valuable. The practice sessions should be short but frequent: three quarter-hour sessions are better than one of half an hour, since fatigue is less likely.

It is difficult to generalize about the length of time needed to become an efficient lipreader. It must depend on a person's age, educational background, intelligence, type of hearing loss, natural aptitude and keenness to learn. Considerable research on what makes for success has been done, but the findings are inconclusive. Lipreading proficiency cannot be attributed to a single factor; natural aptitude, motivation and the possession of a good command of the English language, with a reasonably extensive vocabulary, seem to be particularly important.

LIPREADING IN PRACTICE

In practice the lipreader will benefit from the following suggestions.

If possible, combine lipreading with a hearing aid. Remember that lipreading can substantially increase the effectiveness of a hearing aid and that the converse is also true.

Seek the cooperation of the speaker. Admit to your handicap and avoid bluffing. Do not be afraid to tell the speaker that you need to see his face clearly. Mention that actions such as putting the hand over the mouth, turning away while speaking, or talking and smoking at the same time, make it difficult or impossible for you to lipread. Ask someone who is talking too rapidly to slow down. When shopping, request the salesperson to ring up the prices of the goods on the till so that there will be no misunderstanding. If your lipreading fails ask the speaker to write the message using the Printator device described on page 105.

Take it for granted that you will have to give more conscious attention to what is being said than is necessary for someone with normal hearing. If you find it difficult to grasp the message don't just give up and retreat into your private thoughts. In the early days of lipreading withdrawal is all too easy and is fatal to your future progress. School yourself to concentrate closely. Regard the situation as a challenge to your ability and a test of your powers of observation.

Think ahead. Try to position yourself strategically so that the speaker faces the light and is at a distance (about 6–7 feet) at which you can see the whole of his face without difficulty. Consider beforehand what matters are likely to be talked about in a pending situation. When shopping, for example, you will be conversing about goods and prices; at the doctor's you will be asked to describe your symptoms and so on. In many everyday situations, and especially when you know people well, you will almost be able to guess the questions you will be asked and even the words they will use. Remember, however, that your anticipations may not be realized and thus avoid the embarrassment of answering questions that have never been asked.

Be alert for clues provided by the speaker, his speech and the situation. Observe the speaker's mood as reflected on his face. Is he serious or light-hearted? Does he look at you questioningly? Does he make use of gestures such as shaking his head or pointing? Notice the rhythm of his speech, his pauses and where he puts the emphasis on his words. Use your eyes for clues that may obviate the need for speech. When shopping, for example, look for price tags rather than asking how much an article costs. If you know what subject is being discussed you will deal confidently with homopheneous words: for instance, if you are uncertain whether the speaker said 'bill', 'pill' or 'mill', you can almost without thinking choose the appropriate word from the context. Obviously, if the topic of conversation is the cost of heating and lighting, the right word will probably be 'bill'; 'pill' is appropriate when health or contraception are under discussion, while 'mill' is likely if the topic is the economic history of the cotton industry.

Most people experience some tension when lipreading due to the need to concentrate and the possibility of making a mistake. This tension may reduce your lipreading efficiency. The aim should be to cultivate alertness without being tense. A study of ten deaf lipreaders, skilled in that they were 'able to pick up and carry on normal conversation in a not unusual field at a normal conversational pace', noted that all shared a common characteristic, 'a personality make-up that did not shake under initial failure, or for that matter was not "floored" when things went wrong lip-readingwise. It bespoke basic confidence. Thus, invariably, if the lipreader did not immediately "catch on" the reaction was "Beg pardon?" or "I'm sorry, I didn't get you"—

and so inviting repetition (with perhaps, greater care). A personality given to embarrassment might flinch in a similar situation. We feel that this freedom from reluctance to "speak up" is an invaluable asset to the lip-reader.' (I. Fusfield, *Factors in Lipreading as Determined by the Lipreader*.) As one experienced teacher observed, 'lipreading is 25 per cent skill and 75 per cent confidence'.

SUPPLEMENTING LIPREADING

Given average natural ability, application and confidence, there is no reason why a level of lipreading adequate for most circumstances cannot be achieved, and in practice the uncertainties of lipreading can be partially overcome by four communication methods: manual signs; finger spelling; the Danish mouth-hand system; cued speech.

Manual Signs

Since 1893 most British schools for the deaf have based their teaching of communication on the 'oral system' of speech and lipreading, with the aim of enabling a deaf child to integrate into normal society. Not all pupils succeed in acquiring a command of speech and lipreading sufficient for social adequacy, however, and many welfare officers who are responsible for the deaf in post-school life support the combined system of communication; this supplements lipreading with manual signs and finger spelling. Among the advantages claimed for the combined systems are the following:

(a) It helps overcome the fact that the lipreading ability of many people born deaf is adversely affected by their limited vocabulary and lack of fluency in the use of idiomatic English.
(b) The combined system is more certain than oral communications, and is more useful when it is essential that the deaf person should very accurately comprehend what is said (eg in legal and medical matters).
(c) Signing is a 'natural' method of communication and requires no special effort in learning.
(d) Signing imposes less strain on the visual and mental faculties of deaf people than the use of speech and lipreading exclusively.

The main drawback of the combined system is, of course, that because signing is easier than lipreading a deaf person may come to rely on signs and finger spelling only, and be tempted to give up trying to integrate into the hearing community. Signing is, in any case, disliked and resented by most people who have acquired a profound hearing loss in later life. But readers who are interested are referred to two excellent books, *Conversation with the Deaf* published by the RNID and *The Language of the Silent World*, published by the British Deaf Association.

Finger-Spelling

As shown by Fig 10, finger-spelling simply involves positioning the fingers in 26 different ways to represent the 26 letters of the alphabet. It is possible to learn the 26 positions in less than an hour, but you and your friends and relatives will need considerable practice before messages can be read quickly. The RNID has produced a version of the popular crossword game 'Kan-U-Go' to provide a pleasant way of becoming proficient at finger-spelling. The great objection to finger-spelling, as to signing, is that most people who have become deaf in later life feel that the conspicuous hand movements advertise their disability and cause them to be identified with the born deaf, most of whom have less grasp of language. My view is that this attitude is mistaken. One can understand the reluctance to use manual systems in public, but in the privacy of home, or with close friends, it seems a pity to discard finger-spelling too readily, when it is so easy for everyone to learn.

The Mouth-hand System

This system, in which the speaker uses both mouth and hand to aid the lipreader, was invented by a Danish teacher of the deaf, Georg Forchhammer. It aims to increase the accuracy of lipreading and reduce the strain involved by enabling invisible speech sounds to be more easily identified. Forchhammer recognized that only 30 per cent of all the sounds made in Danish speech could be identified with reasonable certainty. As the vowels belonged to this 30 per cent it was clear that the principal difficulties lay with the consonants. As explained earlier the sounds for p, b and m appear alike on the lips; if you cannot hear them, you can only tell them apart by reference to the context. Fig 11 shows that in the English version of the mouth-hand system, 18 symbols are used to represent 22 consonant sounds. Separate symbols are provided for p, b and

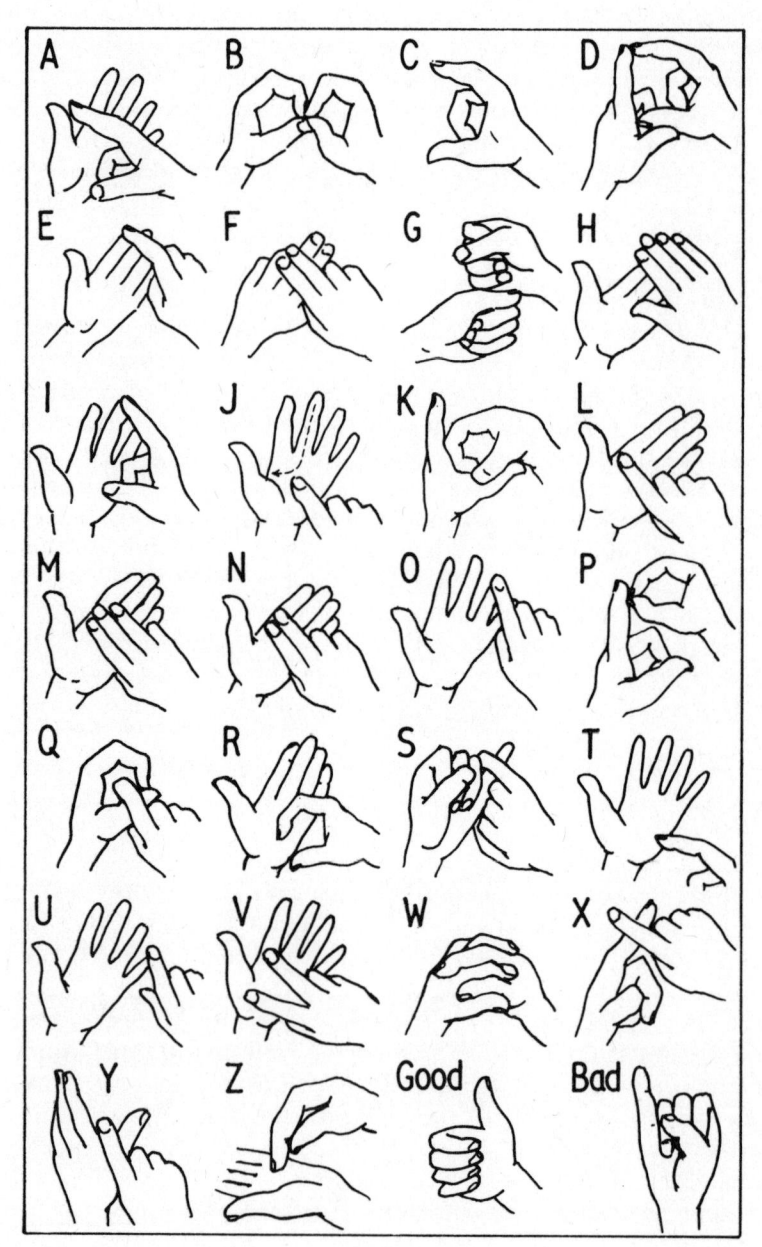

Fig 10

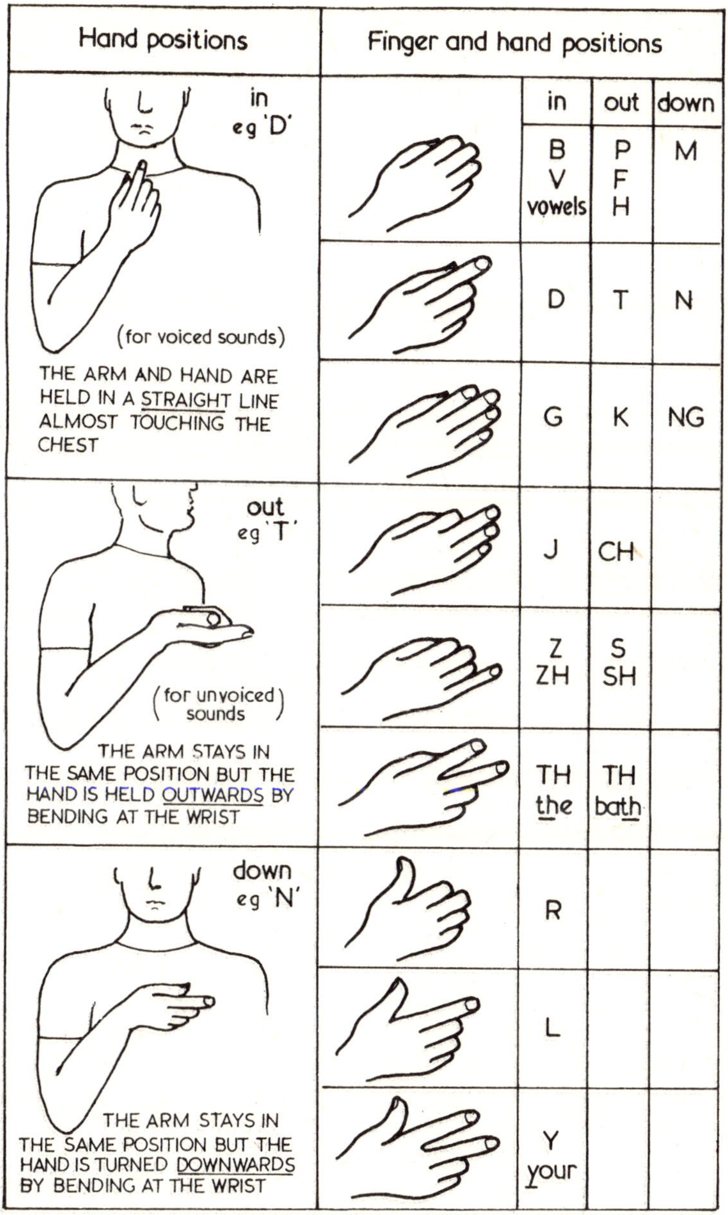

Hand positions	Finger and hand positions			
in eg 'D' (for voiced sounds) THE ARM AND HAND ARE HELD IN A <u>STRAIGHT</u> LINE ALMOST TOUCHING THE CHEST		in	out	down
:::		B V vowels	P F H	M
:::		D	T	N
:::		G	K	NG
out eg 'T' (for unvoiced sounds) THE ARM STAYS IN THE SAME POSITION BUT THE HAND IS HELD <u>OUTWARDS</u> BY BENDING AT THE WRIST		J	CH	
:::		Z ZH	S SH	
:::		TH the	TH ba<u>th</u>	
down eg 'N' THE ARM STAYS IN THE SAME POSITION BUT THE HAND IS TURNED <u>DOWNWARDS</u> BY BENDING AT THE WRIST		R		
:::		L		
:::		Y <u>y</u>our		

Fig 11

m, to cut out the confusion and guesswork.

The various movements are made by one hand positioned under the chin and close to the chest of the speaker. This ensures that both the speaker's mouth and his or her hand can be clearly seen by the lipreader. At the same time, the hand movements are comparatively inconspicuous to other people. Another advantage is that the system can be learnt in about 12 hours and can be used with reasonable confidence after approximately 8 hours' further practice. If you wish to use the system, it is best to seek out a teacher, so that you change incorrect movements before bad habits are formed. This raises a difficulty since teachers are scarce. Fortunately a Mouth-hand System Study Group has been set up to carry on promotional work, and potential students who have difficulty in obtaining tuition should contact the Study Group at the address given in the appendix to this book.

The system is especially useful for people who have suddenly become deaf. It is particularly helpful in a home where at least one member of the family has a profound hearing loss which cannot be overcome with the use of a hearing aid.

Cued Speech

Cued Speech has some similarities to the Danish Mouth-hand System. Both systems aim to support or supplement lipreading, are basically phonetic and involve hand and mouth movements used together. In neither system can a sound be read from the hand movements only. While the mouth-hand system was primarily designed for adults, cued speech was invented (in 1966) to assist deaf or deafened children to acquire the language they have never heard and to develop pronunciation and rhythmic speech. Accordingly, cued speech provides signals for *all* the speech sounds used in normal conversation.

Cued speech has 12 hand shapes or positions. As shown in Fig 12, the 4 hand positions are side, throat, chin and mouth. Consonants are indicated by 8 hand shapes. The person lipreading has to recall which of 25 consonant sounds are associated with a particular hand shape, so cued speech is, in this respect, more complex than the mouth-hand system. Both systems require approximately 20 hours of initial tuition, supplemented by practice.

In London adults can learn cued speech at the City Literary Institute and the Kids National Centre for Cued Speech. The

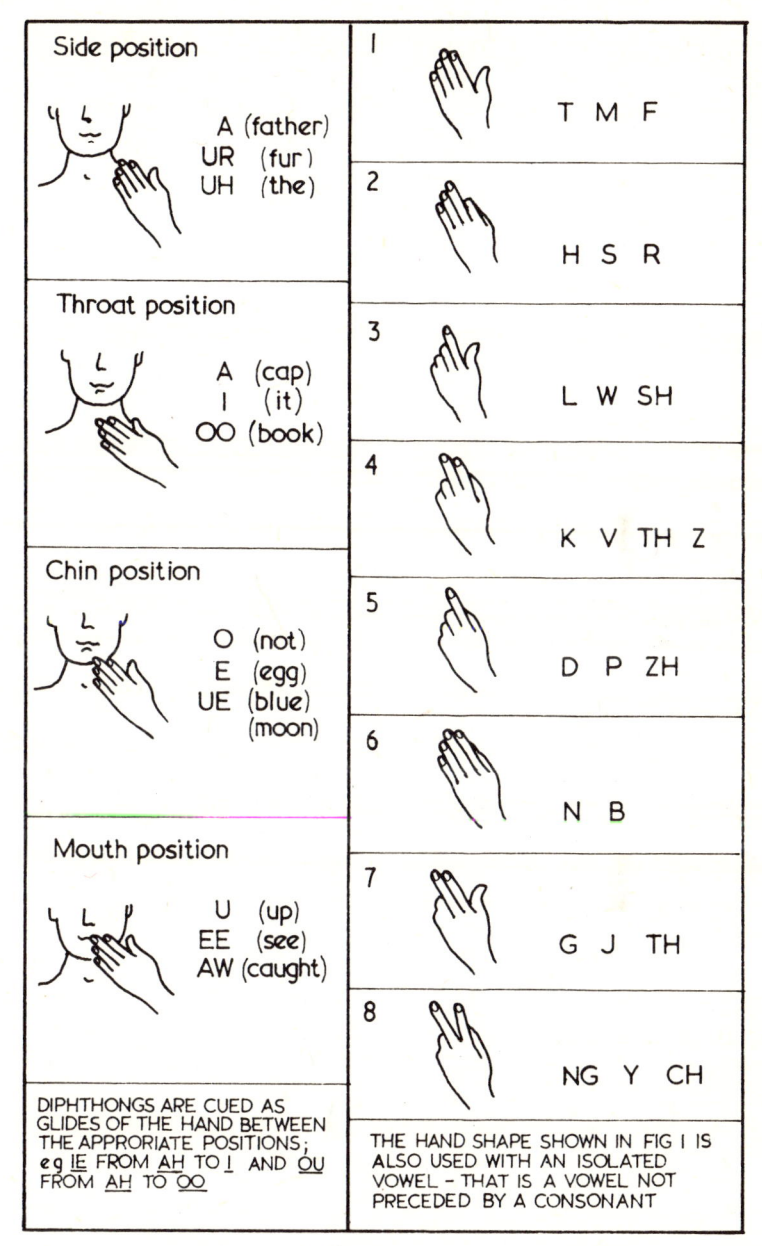

Side position A (father) UR (fur) UH (the)	**1** T M F
	2 H S R
Throat position A (cap) I (it) OO (book)	**3** L W SH
	4 K V TH Z
Chin position O (not) E (egg) UE (blue) (moon)	**5** D P ZH
	6 N B
Mouth position U (up) EE (see) AW (caught)	**7** G J TH
	8 NG Y CH
DIPHTHONGS ARE CUED AS GLIDES OF THE HAND BETWEEN THE APPROPRIATE POSITIONS; eg IE FROM AH TO I AND OU FROM AH TO OO	THE HAND SHAPE SHOWN IN FIG 1 IS ALSO USED WITH AN ISOLATED VOWEL – THAT IS A VOWEL NOT PRECEDED BY A CONSONANT

Fig 12

latter organization was established to inform schools, clinics, local education authorities and, of course, individuals, about the system, so it is to the Centre that any enquiries should be addressed. The Centre has prepared a postal course for would-be students who are unable to obtain class tuition and, in conjunction with the city Literary Institute, awards a Certificate of Proficiency in Cueing and a Diploma in Cued Speech to candidates successful in the required examinations.

AUDITORY TRAINING

The broad aim of auditory training or re-training is to enable a person with impaired hearing to make the best possible use of any residual hearing. This training, for both children and adults, was stimulated by the increased use and availability of electronic hearing aids.

Whether you or any hearing-impaired person you know would benefit from auditory training can be decided only after considering the data obtained from audiometric tests and other information. Audiometric tests will include those for pure tones and speech described earlier in this book. Other factors concerned include the cause, nature and extent of the hearing loss; the age of onset and duration of the impairment; the degree to which the person concerned can compensate for his hearing loss by means of a suitable aid. Where, as with cases of pure conductive loss, a hearing aid enables the user to cope satisfactorily with all normal situations, auditory training is not required. Conversely, where someone has sensorineural loss giving rise to discrimination difficulties, auditory training might be beneficial. Probably the best rough and ready indication for or against the usefulness of auditory training is the person's ability to discriminate between speech sounds.

'Auditory training' covers many components, but a typical programme for adults would include:

Hearing-aid orientation. Advice on the advantages and limitations of monaural and binaural hearing aids; setting the controls for maximum benefit; how to wear the aid neatly and inconspicuously; minor repairs and adjustments.

Listening practice. This may take several forms. It may seek to remedy the inattentiveness and lack of concentration to which hearing-impaired people are prone. It may attempt to improve speech discrimination under both favourable and unfavourable conditions. It may try to improve the person's capacity to localize sounds.

Noise tolerance. Advice as to how noise may be constructively dealt with. This is especially important for people with 'recruitment' problems, when increased volume provided by a hearing aid can lead to diminished discrimination.

Speech improvement. Helping severely deafened adults with longstanding impairments that have resulted in speech and voice deterioration.

Auditory training is usually carried on in small groups but it should be preceded and accompanied by an individual investigation of and attention to the specific needs of each class member.

Successful middle-ear surgery and improved hearing aids have reduced the demand for auditory training and it may be difficult to find either a class or a suitable teacher. As with lipreading, the best plan then is to ascertain how many hearing-impaired people in your area would be willing to take advantage of a course of auditory training should it be available. Armed with this information you can raise the matter at your nearest hearing-aid or audiology clinic or with the local authority Education or Social Services departments. The RNID or the BAHOH may also be able to give useful advice.

9 Employment, Leisure and Family Relationships

Anyone who has a hearing disability knows that it causes a chain reaction of problems affecting every facet of life to some degree. The three important areas in which the effects must be examined and mitigated as far as possible are employment, leisure activities and family relationships.

EMPLOYMENT

The extent to which you are handicapped in your job by a hearing impairment obviously depends on what the job is. In manual occupations, there may be special requirements, such as the need for good hearing to monitor a machine or process, but more often the real difficulty is that to some degree the handicap constitutes a safety hazard. For some jobs adequate hearing is prescribed by regulation. At common law an employer has a duty not only to provide safe conditions of work but also safe fellow-workers and, in certain circumstances, the employment of a hearing-impaired person might be held to be a breach of this requirement. There is also the question of the safety of the hard of hearing person himself. Some employers are reluctant to employ workers who might be at risk because of difficulty in hearing warning signals. However, where safety hazards can be overcome even a severe hearing loss may, in many manual jobs, be a comparatively minor occupational handicap. This is especially so where only a small amount of social interaction is involved and the use of the telephone is not normally required. Captain R. W. Annand, VC, present Chairman of the Vocational Committee of the British Association of the Hard of Hearing, suggests that employers might even find it advantageous to employ the hearing-impaired, for three reasons: such people give greater concentration to the job due to the absence of distractions such as shop-floor gossip; with certain exceptions, eg cases of sensorineural deafness with pronounced recruitment, the hard of hearing may experience less fatigue in noisy working conditions; the hard of hearing have often a highly developed sense of initiative due to the necessity of working out solutions for themselves, thus avoiding the need to ask questions.

With clerical, executive and professional employment, communication difficulties may constitute a severe handicap. Prospects of promotion to more senior posts are often adversely affected for people with poor hearing, as it is in these jobs that communication becomes more important. The allegation is sometimes made that when recruiting or promoting staff, employers 'discriminate' against workers with a hearing handicap: such 'discrimination' is often more apparent than real. An employer, or the personnel officer, is responsible for selecting the best available person for a vacancy. Apart from safety, other factors he must consider are the applicant's potential for re-training and promotion and the reactions of other employees and supervisory staff. For most employers the effect of hearing impairment on job performance is uncertain. Consequently in selecting between two otherwise equal applicants the choice would go against the candidate with a severe loss of hearing. It is unrealistic not to accept the fact that an ambitious hearing-impaired worker does contend with a handicap. If the handicap is to be balanced a high capacity for self-help is required and, sometimes, assistance from government services.

Self-help in Employment

When hearing interferes significantly with employment, the first step is to make a realistic self-appraisal.

What is your expected duration of future working life?

If a hearing loss becomes a handicap in your job at 45 years of age, you have another 15–20 years of working life left. At this age some re-training might be worthwhile. At 55, however, the emphasis should be on retaining present employment.

What is the likely progress of your hearing loss?

Assuming the loss to be irreversible, it is important to have some idea as to whether your hearing will get worse. You may for example be able to use the telephone now, but will you be able to use it in ten years' time? Otologists do not always realize the importance of providing a prognosis that will enable a hearing-impaired person to plan ahead.

Is your present job likely to make hearing worse or give rise to other physical symptoms or mental strain?

Excessive exposure to noise may cause further deterioration in hearing. Trying to cope with the demands of a job in which good hearing is essential may lead to mental strain. These aspects should be discussed with your general practitioner or otologist.

What do you possess in the way of skills, qualifications, vocational experience, interests? To what extent are these marketable?

Consideration of these matters will indicate opportunities for self-employment, re-training or transferring to other work within the same occupation.

What salary is needed to meet fixed expenses such as mortgages, insurances etc? Where can economies be made or income augmented?

Such a financial appraisal is an essential part of any future planning relating to employment.

Such an evaluation will show that age, aptitudes and abilities, together with some knowledge of the likely progress of the disability, present a hearing-impaired person with six possible courses of action over his work: to attempt to retain or improve the existing job; to transfer to alternative work with the same employer; to seek less demanding or more responsible employment elsewhere; to re-train for new work; to become self-employed; to retire prematurely.

Self-employment and premature retirement raise so many individual issues that it is impossible to discuss them here. For the majority of hearing-impaired people the most prudent course of action will be to stay with their present employer. Employers will often make concessions to existing employees that they would not provide for new workers. Furthermore one's colleagues gradually acquire a knowledge of the handicap and can help in many small ways to reduce its impact. It is also possible to get much assistance from the use of aids such as the amplifying telephone handset and the additional earpiece referred to in Chapter 7. Many employers who do not know of these devices might be prepared to install them if asked. Where their use would reduce the strain of work it would pay an employee to meet the cost himself.

If this is not possible, the Employment Services Agency has a scheme for the loan of special aids to registered disabled people who need such equipment to take up or retain employment. The principal object is to provide special aids or attachments needed by the disabled which the non-handicapped would not require to do the same job. The Employment Services Agency will assist in this way when the disabled person cannot meet the cost and the employer is unwilling to do so. Clearly some aids for the hearing-impaired fall into this category, and it may be worth discussing the matter with your local Disablement Resettlement Officer.

Another aid that is useful not merely in employment but in all social situations is the Printator available from the RNID (or sold in stationers). The Printator is essentially a pocket-size notepad, on which messages are written on a celluloid surface which slides in and out. When the celluloid part is pulled out and pushed in again all the writing is erased and new messages can be written.

Anyone who has difficulty in hearing when in a group can seek a strategic seat at meetings from which as many as possible of the other members can be seen, thus facilitating lipreading or supplementing hearing by vision. Normally the best seat for a hearing-impaired person at meetings is next to or opposite the chairman. If you can, with the help of hearing aid and lipreading (which give maximum assistance when used at close quarters), follow most of what the chairman is saying, you will know what subject is under discussion and the point that has been reached on the agenda. It is, moreover, a guide to what is being said by other members of the group, in the same way that some idea can be gleaned of what a caller at the other end of a telephone is saying by listening to the comments of the speaker at the receiving end. In executive jobs a good secretary who can write down telephone messages received and transmit replies, thus acting as both the ears and voice of her boss, is invaluable.

In some cases it may be possible to obtain a transfer within the same organization to a post where good hearing is of less significance. A technical representative who found that his hearing loss was too great a handicap to enable him to continue visiting customers, suggested that his employers should open a market-research department. The suggestion was accepted and he was put in charge. The new department soon demonstrated its usefulness and profitability so that the former representative actually improved his status within the company.

Other examples come readily to mind, such as the deafened bank clerk who was moved from counter work to the supervision of accounts, or the librarian who became an archivist. The point is that thought and initiative will sometimes obviate the need to change the place of employment.

Where such suggestions do not help enough, and you have a lengthy period of working life before retirement, it may be worthwhile to think in terms of re-training. The number of occupations in which hearing impairment may not be too great a handicap is large. I recently asked an employment expert for a list of occupations suitable for deafened or hard-of-hearing adults. After only thirty minutes the following suggestions were made:

Accountancy (financial and cost)	Draughtsmanship
Accountancy machine operation	Farming and market gardening
Archives work	Gardening
Book-binding	Hairdressing
Building trades	Laboratory work
Cartography	Market research
Catering and cookery	Mannequin work or modelling
Chiropody	Painting and decorating
Computer work	Statistical work
Commercial art	Tailoring
Dress designing	Typewriter maintenance
	Typing agency work

Re-training can often take the form of self-training. One can use one's leisure to study for a new occupation by correspondence courses or evening classes. One advantage is that such training is carried on concurrently with normal employment and without the need to leave home or lose income. It can also extend over a longer period and lead to higher qualifications than are available through short intensive courses. High qualities of self-discipline and perseverance are, however, required. To become a member of the Institute of Cost and Management Accountants by part-time study, for example, would take anything from three to six years. One has therefore to start work well in advance of the time when the qualification will be needed.

Government courses are the responsibility of the Training Services Agency. The TSA sponsors residential vocational training for disabled people, including the deaf and hard of hearing, at four colleges: Queen Elizabeth's, Leatherhead; St Loyes, Exeter; Portland, Mansfield; and Finchale, Durham. Candidates are only accepted for training where there is a reasonable prospect that they will qualify for subsequent employment under normal working conditions in the trade they have learned. Courses, which vary in length but in some cases extend over one year, are available at one or more of the above colleges in bench joinery and carpentry, business studies, assistant quantity surveying, cooking, electronic wiring, engineering, draughtsmanship, gardening, instrument craft, industrial electronics, light electro-mechanical fitting, light precision engineering, radio and television servicing, typewriter mechanics, light electrical servicing, storekeeping and watch and clock repair.

In addition to courses of a skilled or semi-skilled variety the TSA may make arrangements for suitably qualified disabled people to attend courses of study leading to the professions.

It is also possible to learn how to do a job by means of a non-residential placement with an employer, or to be sponsored for a course at a College of Further Education. In the latter case the hearing-impaired person would have to show that he was capable of keeping up with students who have normal hearing. Again the first step is to make enquiries through your local Disablement Resettlement Officer.

Government Help in Employment

In any case it is useful to apply for registration as a disabled person under the Disabled Persons (Employment) Acts of 1944 and 1958. Their purpose is to help the handicapped to obtain employment suitable to their capabilities and using their knowledge and skill to the best advantage. The Disabled Persons (Employment) Act of 1944 has been partly repealed by the Employment and Training Act of 1973, but the essentials of the earlier legislation have been retained including the definition of a disabled person as 'One who on account of injury, disease or congenital deformity is substantially handicapped in obtaining or keeping suitable employment'. Also retained are the quota scheme and the arrangements for specialized help through the Disablement Resettlement Officers.

Under the quota scheme every employer with 20 or more workers is required to employ 3 per cent of registered disabled people and to keep records showing the number of such persons on his roll. An employer who is below quota may not without permit from the Disablement Resettlement Officer engage an able-bodied worker or discharge a registered disabled person without reasonable cause. The main functions of Disablement Resettlement Officers is to assist disabled people including, of course, the hearing-impaired, to obtain and keep suitable employment. A DRO can be seen by appointment at any of the Employment Services Agency's job centres or employment offices.

LEISURE

For a hearing-impaired person leisure is not merely freedom from work, it is also a time free from the strain of trying to cope with the demands of an environment in which the assumption is that everyone has normal hearing. Because of this relative freedom from strain there is a danger that a person with a severe hearing loss may tend to do two things. Firstly, as shown in Chapter 6, he or she may withdraw from community life into solitary pursuits. Secondly, the relief at not being involved in the hearing world may be so great that leisure becomes merely a matter of passing the time in activities which provide no permanent satisfaction.

Community Leisure

We spend our leisure in either community or home-centred activities. Community-centred leisure clearly poses problems when we don't hear well, since it normally means a return to the hearing world from which we like to obtain a respite. People with normal ears who urge the hearing-impaired to 'keep in society' often fail to understand that there is nothing that people with auditory handicaps want to do more. The deaf and hard of hearing long for company and conversation with the intensity of blind men longing for sight. What prevents such integration are the difficulties of communication and the attitudes of people with normal hearing—which may include hostility, superiority, impatience and pity, all of which are resented by a sensitive person with a hearing loss. Yet, in the interest of mental health some community life and social contact must be maintained. The motto of the BAHOH is 'Fellowship is life', and the second part of this quotation from William Morris is equally true: 'lack of fellowship is death'.

One way in which a hearing-impaired person may enjoy leisure in a community setting without strain is by becoming a member of a hard-of-hearing club. Over 200 such clubs are affiliated to the BAHOH (from whom a list can be obtained), in addition to a number of youth clubs for people under 35. The club programmes vary widely and, as with similar organizations for any interest-group, reflect the drive and imagination of the club committee and officials. Indoor activities may include dances, whist drives, bingo, games nights, competition evenings, open nights and cinema shows. Outdoor events include visits to local industries, coach trips to seaside resorts and stately homes, rambles, treasure hunts, barbecues and car rallies. One of the greatest pleasures of a club may be the opportunity for a simple conversation over a cup of tea. Membership of a club can also provide an outlet for organizing ability, or for ability in such capacities as treasurer or secretary. If there is no club in your vicinity why not start one? Doing so can be a means of broadening social contacts and using leisure time constructively to help others.

Home-centred Leisure

Obviously leisure at home can be used in endless happy and constructive ways. Three areas where special arrangements have been made for the hearing-impaired, however, are study, painting and watching television plays.

Study. Why not make study your hobby? Such study may be aimed at improving your employability or at gaining a greater understanding of a subject in which you have a particular interest. There are many excellent correspondence colleges which provide guided reading and the assessment of your progress through comments from tutors, and you can study by your own fireside.

Study tends to be more effective when it has an objective, and while many of us dislike examinations there is no doubt that the ability successfully to come through gives a tremendous boost to self-confidence. One of the most enlightened educational innovations of the last decade has been the Open University with its facilities for obtaining a recognized degree by home study. Two sentences from the University's *Guide to Applicants for Undergraduate Courses* are worth quoting: 'Our courses are open to adults irrespective of their age, occupation or previous education and no matter where they live in the United Kingdom.' And 'The Open University student needs no 'A' Level, 'O' Level or other formal educational qualification.'

The Open University remains the only university in the UK to offer systematic help to substantial numbers of hearing-impaired students. Deaf and hard-of-hearing students can participate in the one-week residential summer school which must be attended by every first-year student. Further information can be obtained from the Open University at Walton Hall, Bletchley, Bucks.

By far the largest and most ambitious programme of 'O' and 'A' Level classes arranged specially for the hearing-impaired is provided by the Department of Further Education for the Deaf, set up by the Inner London Education Authority as part of the City Literary Institute. Outside London there is little, if any, special provision.

Painting. Painting gives an opportunity for the personal expression of one's passion for beauty and few hobbies provide such rest to the mind and peace to the spirit. The first step, of course, is to learn how to paint, and art classes are available in most large towns. Painting is particularly suitable for a hearing-impaired person since much of the tuition after the rudiments have been mastered is on an individual basis.

The St James' Art Society for the Deafened was started in 1946 by two artists, one with normal hearing and the other deafened. The society exists 'to help the hearing-impaired to redress their loss of one faculty by increasing their pleasure in another'. In addition to its London activities, which include an annual exhibition of paintings, sculpture, handicrafts and needlework, the society seeks to develop 'country groups' in connection with lipreading classes or hard-of-hearing clubs. The aim of these groups is to help people who, because of distance, are unable to exhibit at the London Exhibition. Members are entitled to join the Society's Artists Magazine Circle; receive copies of the society's Newsletter; receive cards for the society's Exhibition at the Royal Exchange; receive, on request, forms for the Exhibition.

Particulars can be obtained from the Honorary Secretary at the address given in the Appendix to this book.

Watching Television Plays. For many people television is their most enjoyable form of relaxation. Some hearing-impaired people may be inhibited in their viewing because they do not wish to cause inconvenience to their family or neighbours by turning up the volume; others may find it difficult or impossible to hear what speakers are saying irrespective of the loudness of the sound. To assist such viewers the RNID, in conjunction with the BBC, has arranged a play synopsis service. These synopses enable deaf or hard-of-hearing viewers to follow the action of a play even though they cannot hear the speech of the actors. The selection of the plays and the printing of the synopses is the responsibility of the BBC. Should you wish to take advantage of this service you should ask the RNID to add your name to the play synopsis mailing list.

FAMILY RELATIONSHIPS

We need to know much more about the possible effects of a severe hearing impairment on family relationships. To my knowledge no research on this subject has been done either in the UK or the USA, although it has been reported from the USA that the incidence of divorce where both partners are severely deaf is lower than for the general population. Probably the shared knowledge of the consequences of the disability provides mutual understanding. Where, however, either the husband or the wife is handicapped to the extent that normal communication becomes difficult, the effect on the other partner and on members of the family can be significant, and the reasons should be faced.

Hearing impairment restricts the social intercourse of family life. The basis of family life is community. Community, in turn, is dependent on communication. Especially at mealtimes the exchange of news, experiences, gossip and humour helps to cement a bond between members of the family. When one member is unable to join in, he or she may experience a feeling of isolation or rejection. Conversely, the hearing members may feel guilt or embarrassment at 'leaving out' the handicapped person. A marriage may become strained when the whispered intimacies that mean so much between husband and wife become impossible.

Inability to hear can lead to frustration and irritability for both the person affected and other members of the family. The frustration of trying to transmit and receive messages, the necessity of repeating an item several times, or of acting as a second pair of ears, may cause patience to wear thin.

Hearing impairment may make it difficult for partners to develop or maintain common interests. The hearing partner, for example, may enjoy dancing or making new friends. The hearing-impaired partner, however, may find dancing difficult and meeting strangers something of a strain—so he or she will either go to such activities under protest or stay at home. Sheikh and Verney mention a wife who considered her husband to be uninterested because he would not attend parent-teacher meetings, when in reality he was afraid of not hearing what was said and thus appearing stupid. A lady I know resented the fact that her husband would not accompany her to church even though he told her repeatedly that the reason was because he could hear very little of the service.

Hearing impairment may cause a reversal of traditional roles. Thus, where the mother is severely hard of hearing it will be the father who will have to listen for the children and care for them in the night. One hard-of-hearing man remarked 'if we have burglars my wife will have to get up, because I shan't hear them.' Another deafened man resented the fact that his children took their homework to their mother instead of him; they had difficulty in making him understand what they required. A hearing-impaired person's ego can often be bruised by feelings of uselessness, inadequacy and inferiority.

Hearing impairment may give rise to conflict because of the misunderstanding of requests or instructions. Frequently someone who is hard of hearing may protest that he has 'never been told', to which the counter-accusation is that 'you didn't pay attention'.

How these possible causes of friction and breakdown are resolved within a marriage depends primarily on the maturity, understanding and affection of the partners themselves. One man answered the assertion that his severely hard-of-hearing wife 'must be a burden' by quoting Thomas-a-Kempis 'Love takes a burden and makes it no burden'. At the other extreme is the response quoted in a small booklet (Vognsen Sevend, *Hearing Tactics*) issued by the Danish State Hearing Institute (English edition by the National Council of Health Education): 'Marriage problems? My answer to this must be "Yes". To me it was simply a catastrophe. My husband thought it was horrible to have a hearing-impaired wife. He thought I was a millstone round his neck. When I realised I could sink no deeper or get no worse I had my divorce.'

There is a great need for short intensive courses to help normal-hearing people become orientated to the problems of the severely hard of hearing and deafened. A two-week residential course is provided by the Link Centre for Deafened People, at Eastbourne. It aims to help people handicapped by sudden, severe or total deafness or 'those who suffer severe irreversible or encroaching deafness together with members of their family'. For those attending it provides a tailor-made programme, which may include intensive help with communication skills, employment questions and similar problems. Part or all of the cost of the course may be met by the Social Services Department of the towns in which the course members reside.

Factors that help in ensuring that hearing impairment affecting one partner has the minimum effect on family relationships are the following.

Emotional security. A hearing-impaired person who is loved, respected and accepted will be less likely to succumb to feelings of inferiority and hopelessness, and the tension arising from frustration will be less.

A positive self-concept. The hearing-impaired person must be encouraged to play as full a part as possible in home activities. He or she must be consulted on domestic decisions and never bypassed because of the difficulties of communication.

Communication skills. Both the hearing-impaired person and members of the family should do everything possible to learn lipreading, and such aids to lipreading as Cued Speech or the Danish Mouth-Hand system. The greater the mastery of these skills, the more the hard-of-hearing person will be included in the family circle.

Communication aids. The various devices such as flashing doorbells and vibrators described in Chapter 6 can take away much frustration and uncertainty.

Finally, as suggested in Chapter 5, the person with hearing loss must be prepared to develop empathy. Such empathy will help to stifle self-pity and lead to an awareness that a disability causes problems not only for himself or herself but for all members of the family. He should seek not only to be understood but also to understand.

10 Statutory and Voluntary Services for People with Impaired Hearing

The purpose of this final chapter is to give an outline of the scope and development of the statutory services for the hearing impaired, and the main national voluntary organizations and their activities.

STATUTORY SERVICES

The National Assistance Act 1948

Statutory recognition to adults with a hearing impairment was given for the first time in Section 29 of the National Assistance Act 1948. It empowered the then County and County Borough Councils to make arrangements for: 'Promoting the welfare of persons who are blind, deaf or dumb and other persons who are substantially handicapped by illness, injury and congenital deformity and such other disabilities as may be described by the Minister.'

It is important to note that the wording of the Act is 'deaf *or* dumb' not 'deaf *and* dumb' and the word 'deaf' is therefore a generic term covering all categories of hearing impairment. In 1948 the local authorities had discretion to provide services for categories of handicapped persons other than the blind and it was not until 1960 that the Minister directed local authorities to exercise their powers with reference to the deaf or dumb.

Meanwhile, in 1951, the Minister had issued a Circular (32/51) setting out a model scheme detailing the services that a local authority must or might provide for the deaf or dumb. The circular has still not been withdrawn, so it indicates the kind of services you can enquire about. The model scheme was applicable to both the deaf and the hard of hearing and the Minister stated that he would be reluctant to approve schemes submitted by local authorites unless they included arrangements for the following services.

Assistance to deaf or dumb persons to overcome the effects of their disabilities and to obtain treatment.
An advisory service on personal and other problems.
Encouragement to deaf or dumb persons to take part in social activities.
Visitation by voluntary workers.

In the Minister's model scheme, the following services *could* be provided.

Provision of practical assistance in the home.
Provision of assistance in obtaining wireless, library and other recreational facilities.
Provision of lectures, games and other recreational facilities in social centres by way of outings, etc.
Provision of, or arranging for, special religious services.
Provision of travelling facilities so that deaf or dumb persons can take advantage of the service provided.
Helping deaf or dumb persons to take holidays at holiday homes.
Provision of social centres or holiday homes.

Circular 32/51 also required local authorities to keep a register of handicapped persons who applied for help. For the hearing-impaired this register, as revised in 1961, was to subdivide into the following three categories, according to the person's *present* condition and needs rather than according to the *origin* of his disability.

Deaf without speech: those who have no useful hearing and whose normal method of communication is by signs, finger spelling or writing.

Deaf with speech: those who (even with a hearing aid) have little or no useful hearing but whose normal method of communication is by speech and lipreading.

Hard of hearing: those who (with or without a hearing aid) have some useful hearing and whose normal method of communication is by speech, listening and lipreading.

Under the Local Government Act 1972 (Section 195(3)) schemes relative to the welfare of handicapped persons approved in the National Assistance Act may pass to our new local authorities.

Especially since the passing of the Local Authority Social Services Act an increasing number of local authorities have appointed their own welfare officers for the hearing-impaired and are taking over responsibility either wholly or in part from the voluntary societies. There are still wide variations in the range and quality of services provided by the Social Services Departments. Some authorities do far too little for the deafened and hard of hearing. Others, such as the Lancashire County Council, provide outstanding service. In Lancashire such services are based on two fundamental principles. Firstly, *all* hearing-impaired people in the county are to be helped. This means the recognition that in addition to the deaf without speech, services must be provided for such groups as the deaf with speech, the deaf-blind, deaf children and their families, the traumatically deafened and the hard of hearing. Secondly, *all* the service personnel in the Social Services Department should be encouraged to offer their skills and services to the hearing-impaired, using the authority's social-worker adviser for the deaf and his staff when specialized assistance is required.

Overall, the last two decades have witnessed a great improvement in most areas in the scope and quality of welfare work for the hearing-impaired. If, therefore, you or your relative or friend have problems of any kind arising from a hearing handicap you should not be diffident about contacting the Social Services Department of your local authority. This carries no stigma and in the overwhelming majority of cases expert advice and constructive help is given.

The Chronically Sick and Disabled Persons Act

Hearing-impaired people may also be eligible for assistance under the terms of this Act, Section 2 of which requires a local authority Social Services Department, when it is satisfied of the necessity to do so, to provide or give assistance to handicapped persons to obtain all or any of the following services: practical assistance in the home; wireless, television, library or similar recreational facilities in the home; recreational and travelling facilities outside the home and assistance in taking advantage of educational facilities; support in minimizing the social and personal consequence of illness and disability to individuals and families; assistance in carrying out adaptations to the home or provision of additional facilities to secure greater safety, comfort or convenience; facilitating the taking of holidays; meals at home or elsewhere; telephone and any special equipment necessary for its use.

Sections 1 and 2 of the Act also state that: 'it shall be the duty of every local authority having functions under Section 29 of the

National Assistance Act to inform themselves of the number of persons to whom that section applies within their area and of the need for the making by the authority arrangements under that section for such persons.'

In June 1976, the Secretary of State for Social Services announced that a new Institute was being established by the Medical Research Council with the aim of providing a base for a multi-disciplinary research effort in the field of hearing impairment. The first Director of the Institute started work at the beginning of 1977.

Government Policy for the Hearing Impaired

This is under regular review. The 'Panel of Four Principal National Organizations for the Hearing Impaired' meets regularly with the Secretary of State for the Social Services. The Department of Health & Social Security has a social work officer specializing in hearing impairment, and an Advisory Committee on Services for the Hearing Impaired on which there is a wide range of expertise. The Medical Research Council has already done much useful work, and activity will be continued through the new Institute of Hearing Research. Through their advisory machinery and contacts with the voluntary organizations, government departments are aware that much research needs to be done. A recent report of the Department of Health & Social Security gives encouragement for the future: 'It has been accepted that service provision for the deaf and hard of hearing should be given some priority. The main objectives are to improve the standards in audiology departments and hearing-aid centres by expansion of staff and facilities, including facilities for follow-up and rehabilitation of patients provided with hearing aids.'

NATIONAL VOLUNTARY ORGANIZATIONS

Reference has been made earlier in this chapter to the 'Panel of Four Principal National Organizations for the Hearing Impaired'. These organizations comprise The British Association of the Hard of Hearing; The British Deaf Association; The National Deaf Children's Society and The Royal National Institute for the Deaf. Readers of this book will be particularly interested in the BAHOH and the RNID.

The British Association of the Hard of Hearing

The BAHOH founded in 1947 is the national body for those who have become wholly or partially deaf usually in post-school life. Its members, therefore, have normal speech and education and employ hearing aids and lipreading as their means of communication. The Association offers the hard of hearing a range of services, especially facilities for social activities and assistance with personal problems. Social activities are based primarily on the over 200 hard-of-hearing clubs located throughout the country. The Association arranges holidays, both at home and abroad, social gatherings or rallies and weekend courses of lectures and recreational work such as pottery, basketwork etc. Pen-circles are also organized for the lonely or housebound and people who live too far from a club.

Help with personal problems includes advice on hearing aids and employment. Employment advice can be obtained from an experienced vocational officer. In addition, the Association has a team of voluntary social-service advisers who can visit individuals to discuss problems and suggest further sources of help. Like all the national organisations for the hearing impaired, the BAHOH maintains close relationships with appropriate government departments to whom complaints and other enquiries can be rapidly conveyed.

The BAHOH can be joined in one of two ways. Firstly, membership of an affiliated hard-of-hearing club carries automatic BAHOH membership. Secondly, it is possible for non-club members to become general members. The magazine of the Association, published quarterly, is *Hark*.

The British Deaf Association

The BDA, founded in 1890 as the British Deaf and Dumb Association, offers its services to all hearing-impaired people although it is primarily the national organization for those born with severe deafness or those deafened in childhood. There are about 160 BDA branches, most of them associated with local voluntary centres for adult deaf people. The BDA undertakes for the deaf many of the activities provided by the BAHOH for the heard of hearing. It has an outstanding youth and further-education service which gives grants for educational purposes and organises residential courses for both adults and young people. A home for elderly deaf people is maintained. The Association is Great Britain's representative to the World

Federation of the Deaf and studies current international developments in health, education and welfare. The BDA has initiated or participated in several useful surveys dealing with various aspects of the needs of deaf people. Individuals can join the BDA—write to the secretary. The journal of the Association, published bi-monthly, is *The British Deaf News*.

The National Deaf Children's Society

The NDCS was formed in 1944 and is the national organisation concerned with deaf children. The word 'deaf' in the title is used in its widest sense, applying to all children whose hearing impairment constitutes a handicap. The Society's purpose is to see that children born deaf, or who became deaf at an early age, are enabled to live fulfilling lives. It offers help with the home environment, educational and medical facilities.

The NDCS works through over fifty regional associations some of which have a number of branches. The society welcomes as members, parents, teachers of the deaf, otologists, social workers with deaf people and all active well wishers of deaf children. The NDCS journal published quarterly is *Talk*.

The Royal National Institute for the Deaf

The RNID is the only national body dealing with all aspects of hearing impairment. Through its influential contacts with government departments and pressure-group activities, it promotes and protects the interests of all the deaf and hard of hearing. It also acts as a co-ordinating agency for organizations interested in various aspects of hearing impairment. The Institute's Council includes representatives from medicine, education and the social services, as well as people with other special interests relating to deafness. Representatives of appropriate government departments attend the Institute's council meetings as observers.

Many of the services offered by the RNID have already been mentioned. Anyone requiring advice or assistance may call at or write to the Institute, where the query will receive sympathetic, expert and constructive attention.

The work of the Institute, as it affects the individual deaf or hard of hearing person or others concerned with the handicap, is divided into four main sections.

Library and information services
The library comprises the most comprehensive collection of books and journals in the world on audiology and associated fields.

Publications
A bi-monthly magazine *Hearing* and also a range of publications relating to hearing impairment.

Social services
Advice, support and information are provided on personal, family and employment problems arising from hearing impairment.

Scientific and technical
The Institute maintains laboratories in London and Glasgow; research is undertaken into hearing aids, other special aids to hearing and educational equipment. Of special interest to readers of this book is the Hearing Aid Advisory Service referred to in Chapter 7.

The Institute also maintains a number of residential centres. These include a school for maladjusted deaf and partially hearing children; a training centre for maladjusted deaf young men; a hostel for deaf young men who are in employment; and homes where elderly deaf people can be cared for in an environment where their difficulties are understood.

Membership of the Institute, which gives the right to vote at elections to the Council and to receive a copy of *Hearing*, requires the payment of a minimum annual subscription (at present £2.50).

Appendix I

Hearing Aid Council

CODE OF PRACTICE

Whereas the terms of the following Code of Trade Practice have been approved in writing by the Secretary of State for Trade and Industry:

Now, therefore, the Hearing Aid Council, acting pursuant to Section 1 (3) of the Hearing Aid Council Act 1968 (hereinafter referred to as 'the Act'), hereby prescribe the following code of trade practice for adoption by persons registered as dispensers of hearing aids under the Act and by persons employing such dispensers:

Dispensers

1. Dispensers shall not indicate the fact that they are registered under the Act by means of any written representation involving the use of words other than 'registered under the Hearing Aid Council Act 1968'.

2. Where those words are employed in an advertisement or promotional literature they shall be accompanied by a statement of the fact that this code of practice is available to any person on request and such a copy shall be made available to anyone requesting it.

3. Dispensers shall maintain at all times a high standard of ethical conduct in the operation of their practice.

4. Dispensers shall at all times give the best possible advice they can to their clients regarding hearing aids and their use.

5. Dispensers shall, where appropriate, make it known to their clients that a hearing aid may not necessarily be of benefit.

6. Dispensers who are not medically qualified shall advise a client to seek medical advice, if he has not already done so, if it appears that the client has been exposed to loud noise in his work or elsewhere or if the client complains of or shows any of the following:-

(a) excessive wax in the ear (whether revealed by examination prior to taking an ear impression or otherwise);
(b) discharge from the ear;
(c) dizziness or giddiness (vertigo);
(d) earache;
(e) deafness only of short duration or of sudden onset;

(f) unilateral perceptive deafness;
(g) conductive hearing loss;
(h) tinnitus (ringing or other noises in the ear or ears).

7. Dispensers who are not medically qualified shall not:-
   (a) represent themselves in any way as being so qualified;
   (b) practise any form of medical or surgical treatment for deafness;
   (c) at any time assume the status of one having surgical or medical knowledge;
   (d) advertise that they are in a position to cure any human failing or physical ill.

8. Dispensers shall not describe themselves as consultants, or specialists, or audiologists unless immediately preceded by the words 'Hearing Aid'.

9. Dispensers shall not designate any premises as a Clinic or Institute.

10. Dispensers shall not interview any potential client at his or her home with regard to the possible provision of a hearing aid unless requested to do so by the client, or unless such client has already been in communication with the dispenser or his employer and, having been given reasonable opportunity, has not indicated objection to such visit.

11. (i) A dispenser must have available for use at every consultation the following equipment:-
   (a) A pure tone audiometer (I.E.C. Publication 177 'Pure tone audiometers for general diagnostic purposes'), regularly calibrated to an acceptable standard (B.S. 2497 Parts 1 to 4), and which contains the facilities for both air and bone conduction audiometry with masking.
   (b) An auriscope and specula together with facilities for cleaning them.
   (c) Suitable aural impression material and associated equipment.
   (d) A range of air conduction (ear-level and body-worn) hearing aids, and of bone conduction hearing aids.

   (ii) A dispenser must also be able to arrange speech audiometry when required.

12. Unless a pure tone audiogram taken within the previous two months by, or under the supervision of an ear, nose and throat specialist is available to the dispenser at the time of consultation, appropriate air conduction and bone conduction audiometry must be carried out, with the use of masking where necessary.

13. Before providing or effecting the supply of a hearing aid or before the client has entered into any commitment if this should be later, dispensers shall provide the client in writing with details of:-

- (i) the conditions relating to any trial, whether free or otherwise;
- (ii) the terms of any guarantee;
- (iii) the service arrangements available for the hearing aid; and
- (iv) the cash price, if any, for the hearing aid and any additional charges and details of any alternative terms or rental terms offered by him to that client.

14. Dispensers shall not take part directly or indirectly in the making of survey enquiries by personal contact or telephone from members of the public regarding deafness or the sale of hearing aids with a view to securing business.

15. Dispensers shall be responsible for the work of any person whose name has been notified to the Registrar in accordance with the provisions of section 3 (1) (a) (ii) of the Act and who is operating under their supervision. They shall also ensure that any such person complies with the code of practice for dispensers set out in paragraphs 1 to 14 above.

16. Dispensers who are self-employed or who carry on business in partnership with other dispensers shall comply with the code of practice set out in the preceding paragraphs and also with that part of the code for employers as is set out in paragraphs 23, 24 and 25 below.

17. The due date by which every dispenser must comply with Rules 11 and 12 is to be 1st December, 1974.

(Reproduced by permission of the Hearing Aid Council)

Appendix II
Organisations useful to people with impaired hearing

Advertising Standards Authority.
   Director and Secretary: Peter Thomson, 15-17 Ridgmount Street, London WC1E 7AW.
British Association of the Hard of Hearing.
   Secretary General: C. H. Mardell, MBE, 16 Park Street, Windsor, Berks. SL3 1LU.
British Deaf Association.
   General Secretary: A. B. Hayhurst, MBE, 38 Victoria Place, Carlisle, CA1 1EX.
City Literary Institute—Centre for the Deaf.
   Head of Centre: K. S. Pegg, CTD, Keeley House, Keeley Street, London WC2.
Hearing Aid Council.
   Registrar: D. Reid, 226 City Road, Old Street, London EC1V 2PP.
Hearing Aid Industry Association.
   Secretary: Mervin Thomas, Broadway House, The Broadway, London SW19 1RL.
Institute of Hearing Research.
   Director General: Professor Mark Haggard, Department of Medicine, University of Nottingham.
The Link Centre for Deafened People.
   Director: Miss R. F. McCall, c/o Princess Alice Memorial Hospital, Eastbourne, Sussex, BN2 12AX.
Mouth-Hand System Study Group.
   Chairman: John Willoughby, 20 Connaught Road, St Albans, Herts, AL3 5RX.
National Centre for Cued Speech.
   Principal: Mrs June P. Dixon, 17 Sedlescombe Road, London SW6 1RE.
National Deaf Children's Society.
   Director: Mrs Betty Scott-Ashworth, 31 Gloucester Place, London W1H 4EA.
Open University.
   Undergraduate Admissions: PO Box 48, Milton Keynes, MK7 6AB.

Royal National Institute for the Deaf.
  Secretary-General: Roger Sydenham, 105 Gower Street, London WC1 6AH.
St James Art Society for the Deafened.
  Hon Secretary: Miss A. C. Pollock, Quendon Cottage, Quendon, Nr Saffron Walden, Essex.
Society of Hearing-Aid Audiologists.
  Secretary: P. A. Wells, 54 Croham Manor Road, South Croydon, Surrey, CR2 7BE.

Acknowledgements

In writing the book I have, to adapt a phrase of Charles Reade's, 'filled my bucket from many taps'. While the source of all quotations and illustrations has been acknowledged in the text it would be impracticable to mention by name all those who have given assistance or advice.

There are, however, seven people to whom I am especially grateful. My debt to Miss Mary Plackett, the Librarian of the RNID, who has dealt patiently, courteously and competently with many requests for information cannot be adequately expressed in words. I am also indebted to Mr C. H. Mardell, Secretary General of the British Association of the Hard of Hearing; Dr T. J. Watson, Reader in the Department of Audiology and the Education of the Deaf in the University of Manchester; Mr M. C. Martin of the RNID who read in draft part of Chapter 7; Miss A. Samuell, Educational Audiologist to the St Helens Borough Council, and the Medical Adviser to the RNID journal *Hearing*, made some invaluable comments in connection with Chapters 2 and 4.

I would also place on record my appreciation of the kindness of the Editor of *Hearing* for permission to use autobiographical material that first appeared in his magazine under the title of 'Necessity to Glorious Gain'.

Index

Adler, A., 64-5
Advertising Standards Authority, 80
aids: 84-6
   amplifying telephone handset, 86,
   extension bells, 86;
   hearing (*see* hearing aids)
   lamp signals, 86-7
   radio and television, 85
   Tonecaller or Trimphone, 86
   visual and other signals, 87
   watch receiver, 86
Annand, R. W., 102
Ashley, Jack, 57
audiograms: 33
   interpretation of, 38, 40-4
audiometers and audiometry, 31-40
   advantages of audiometry, 48;
   Békésy audiometer, 32;
   control on audiometer, 31-2,
   pure tone audiometry, 34-5;
   speech audiometry, 35-7
auditory training, 100-1

Békésy, G. von, 32
Bell, A. G., 31, 66
Boothroyd A., 36
British Association of the Hard of
   Hearing, 109, 118
British Deaf Association, 118
Burchett, J. H., 88

Carhart Notch, 40
cholesteatoma, 21
Chronically Sick and Disabled Persons
   Act, 116-17
City Literacy Institute, 91, 110
conductive hearing loss, 18-22
cued speech, 98-100

Danish mouth-hand system, 95-8
deaf, distinguished from hard of
   hearing, 5-7
decibels, 29-31
Disabled Persons Employment Act,
   107-8

ear: 12, 16
   anatomy, 12, 17;
   moulds, 71-2;
   trumpets and tubes, 66
**emotional and behavioural results of
hearing loss**: 56-65
   bluffing, 9, 57, 58, 61-2;
   depression, 57-9;
   fear, 56-7;
   frustration, 59-60;
   inferiority, 61, 64-5;
   withdrawal, 9, 57
employment, 102-8
Evans, J. D., 6
Ewing, A. and E. C., 90

family relationships, 111-14
fenestration operation, 51
finger spelling, 95
Forchammer, G., 98
Fry, D. B., 36
Fusfield, I., 94

Gerber, S. E., 17
glue ear, 21
Goffman, M. A., 61
Goldstein, M. A., 66
government policy for the hearing
   impaired, 117

hearing aid(s): 66-84
   all-in-the-ear, 69;
   batteries, 70-1;
   behind-the-ear, 68;
   binaural, 69;
   bodyworn, 67;
   commercial, 74-8;
   components, 69-71;
   controls, 72-3;
   cost, 75-7;
   ear-level, 67-8;
   exhibitions, 78-80;
   faults, 82-4;
   maintenance, 82;
   National Health, 73-4;
   rental, 76-7;
   spectacle, 68-9;
   types, 66;
   use of, 81-2
Hearing Aid Council, 79-80, 121-3

Hearing Aid Council Act, 79
hearing, binaural, 16-17
hearing loss: 18-26, 27, 44
   causes of, 18-26
   measurement of, 27-44;
   stapedectomy, 51-4;
   stapes mobilisation, 51-2

Institute of Hearing Research, 117

Jeffers and Barley, 89

Keller, H., 35

lipreading: 87-101
   advantages, 89-90;
   basis of, 87-9;
   learning, 90-2;
   limitations of, 89;
   practice of, 92-4;
   supplementing, 94-101
Leisure: 108-11
   Community centres, 108-9;
   home centred, 109-10;
   Link Centre for Deafened People, 113

manual signs, 94-5
Mardell, C. H., 26
Mawson, S. R., 38
Ménière's disease, 23-4, 54, 55
Meyerson, L., 57-8
Morris, William, 109
myringoplasty, 50
myringotomy, 49

National Assistance Act, 114-15
National Deaf Childrens' Society, 119
Newby, H. A., 33
Niebuhr, R., 65

Open University, 110
ossicyloplasty, 50
otitis-media, 19, 20-1, 50
otologist consulting, 45-6
otosclerosis, 21, 22, 51-4

painting, 110-11

'Panel of Four', 117
Pavitt, L., 79
presbyacusis, 24-5

Ramsdell, D. A., 59
recruitment, 37, 44, 81
Rosen, S., 25, 51
Royal National Institute for the Deaf, 119-20
   battery tester, 71,
   Hearing Aid Advisory Service, 79,
   Kan-U-Go game, 95,
   Medresco purse, 82,
   play synopsis service, 111,
   printator, 105;
   publications, 67, 71, 85, 95

St James' Art Society, 110
senservineural loss, 22-5
   audiograms in, 42-4
Sheikh, 84
social attitudes to hearing impaired, 60-2
sound, nature of, 27-9
speech reading (*see* lipreading)
spondee words, 35
Statistics: 51-2
   deaf, 5-7;
   hard-of-hearing, 5-7
study as a hobby, 109-10
syringing, 45

Thomas-à-Kempis, 113
tinnitus, 25-6
Topophone, 17
Training Services Agency, 107
tuning fork tests: 47-8
   Rinne, 47;
   Schwabach, 48;
   Weber, 47
tympanoplasty, 50

Verney, A., 84
vertigo, 54-5
Vognsen, S., 113

Warfield, F., 61
Wilde, W., 50